The Angel's

By

Altaf Hussain

How I Overcame Cancer the Natural Way

Memoirs of an International Lawyer

First published 2020.

Altaf Hussain, London

Disclaimer

The contents of this book reflect the author's personal experiences. This book is not meant to be used, nor should it be used, to diagnose or treat any medical condition. The material in this book relates to the author's own experiences of cancer, and the book is in no way intended to suggest any cure or treatment for cancer, or any other medical condition of any kind. For any diagnosis or treatment of any medical issue we strongly advise that readers consult their own doctor or physician. Neither the author nor the publisher is responsible for any medical or health needs from which the reader, or any person they know, may suffer. They are not liable for any damages or negative consequences for any treatment, action, application or preparation used by any person, or their associates, who read this book.

This book is sold with the understanding that neither the publisher nor the author is either engaged, or qualified, to offer any type of medical advice. Neither the author nor the publisher shall be liable for any physical, psychological, emotional, financial or commercial damages of any kind. Our views and rights are the same: the reader and their associates are responsible for their own choices, actions and consequences.

About the Author

Solicitor and International Lawyer Altaf Hussain was born in 1977, he was educated at King Edward's Grammar School and Birmingham City University. He established Addison Aaron in 2009, England's leading boutique international law firm.

Addison Aaron has dealt with contentious and complex issues spanning more than twenty-five jurisdictions. The firm has won multiple awards from The Law Society of England and Wales.

When he was diagnosed with cancer in 2011, Altaf continued to work full time and decided to decline chemotherapy and instead opted to treat himself naturally with diet.

Altaf is an avid sportsman, he lives in England with his wife.

'Let food be your medicine and medicine be food.' – Hippocrates the father of medicine

'The seed is meat for you.' – The Holy Bible

The Prophet Mohammed (PBUH) said: *'For every disease there is a medicine, and if that medicine is applied to the disease, he will recover by Allah's leave.'*

He also said: *'Allah has not sent down any disease but he has also sent down the cure; the one who knows it, knows it, and the one who does not know it, does not know it.'*

With thanks for the love and support of my family and friends.

Contents

Introduction

11th September 2013

Letter from the Heartlands hospital to my GP.

From my Consultant Haematology Team

Mr Hussain is really very well. His weight is stable, and he remains fit and active. Examination was unremarkable. There is no clinical evidence of any progression of his disease, and as you know we are happy to have a policy of close observation at the moment.

Can anything offer us greater wealth than our health? The richest person in the world cannot buy a new body or find a cure for cancer.

The pages that follow are memoirs; this is not an autobiography. It is a series of recollections around the things that are important to me. I suppose that most people can divide their lives into three main interwoven parts; their family and loved ones, their social lives and their career. I touch on all of these in this book, and with regards to my career, I hope that I offer some really interesting and useful anecdotes and experience

8

of being a successful international lawyer. I am the co-founder and chairman of Addison Aaron. This is probably the most successful boutique international law firm in the country; there are no hard and fast criteria which I can use to reach that conclusion, admittedly, but I think (as the book will show) I have a number of foundations upon which I can make such a claim.

I will share some of the details of the interesting cases of which I have been a part, but of course, as a professional, I can assure readers that this is not a 'kiss and tell' memoir; the identity of my clients remain confidential.

As I have said, most of us can broadly divide our lives in three main departments. Some people, though, have a fourth. For a significant minority of us, our health becomes a major factor throughout our lives. I was just a young man, little more than a boy, when I was diagnosed with cancer for the first time. I was a successful lawyer, newly married and my own fledgling firm when it hit me for the second. I have experienced the traditional approach to dealing with cancer – chemotherapy. I have also experimented with my own, diet based, attempt to tackle the disease. Nine years after my second bout, I am still here, still active, still fit and still healthy.

I have wanted to share my experiences for a while now. At this point I should add that this book does not offer a cure for cancer, nor does it provide advice for the treatment of cancer. It simply tells of my experiences; the medical ones and the ones based on what I consumed. It is an opportunity to summarise and share the knowledge I acquired under the grave circumstances in which I found myself. Twice. I will describe how I treated myself for cancer and how I continue to do so, in my best attempts to prevent the disease visiting me for a third time.

This book is also not an attempt to advise on cancer – there are professionals in every hospital whose knowledge, experience and know-how far, far exceeds mine. This is simply an account of what I did, why I did it and the experience of the disease I live through.

I am sharing my story, my understanding and my struggles to give hope and to evidence that miracles can happen. In our darkest hours in the end most of us seek refuge in the Lord, or our own spiritual equivalent. We can help ourselves if we read, seek knowledge and then take action.

I also consider the mental and emotional impacts of cancer. They are as frightening and debilitating as the physical ones. However, I hope that this book will show that they can be faced, challenged and defeated.

One of the reasons I have been keen to include some of my experiences as a lawyer, is I do feel that the attitude to adversity I found myself demonstrating during my cancer events, is similar to the one I adopt in legal matters. I find that a bullish approach is vital, this approach requires tremendous amount of energy, consideration, backbone and thought. The dominant question is always 'How can I win?' Positivity to the fore. Yet that positivity is built on realism. Nothing is guaranteed. Positivity makes a difference, but no result is certain. Not in life, not in the law courts, not in the fight against cancer. Yes, it is important to be confident, determined, proactive and decisive. But always bringing along humility as their companion. I do believe that if I can do it, then anybody can do it. Please take that confidence whether you are a cancer sufferer, a friend or family of a victim, a lawyer setting out on a career or a reader who just wants to take in another person's perspective on living life to the max, if occasionally on the edge.

I believe in looking forward, being courageous, having outrageous personal goals, but I reiterate that this book is a memoir, it is not a manual offering legal or medical advice; the way I treated myself has not been scientifically proven as a solution for, or an approach towards, curing cancer. Further, my book is in no way meant to advise people with cancer as to how they should treat themselves. I am just sharing my experiences.

Given everything said in the paragraphs above, it is a reasonable question to ask, 'Why now?' I am nine years past my last bout of cancer, and although I still have worries, still take close care of my diet, I have moved on. But I wrote this preface on April 18th, 2020. The world was in the grip of an unprecedented global lockdown. On this day, it had been in my plans to fly to Spain with my mates Bob, Shyfa and Uncle Shahed. But flights had been cancelled. We had planned this getaway for months, and instead of embarking on an enjoyable break, I was, like almost the entirety of the remainder of the UK, stuck at home.

It seemed to me that there were parallels between my experience, shared with much of the world, of lockdown thanks to Covid 19, and the personal, internal lockdown I experienced from cancer. Something shared with plenty of others, but not a majority of people. But then I began to think. To wonder about the disease. It hit me that the impact of cancer not only strikes at people who develop the disease, but also an ever-widening circle of their family, friends and colleagues. If cancer is the stone that strikes the heart of the pond, its ripples spread remorselessly outwards from this central point.

Of course, we are learning all of the time about Covid 19; we are also learning of the chaos at the heart of Governments across the world as they try to deal

12

with the virus. We know that Boris Johnson had been elected Prime Minister for barely three months when he instilled the most dramatic restrictions on personal liberty in the history of the nation. Including two world wars. We know that the advice from the scientific community on which he relied led to his actions, but also now that these scientists were very much in the dark about the disease. As oncologists often still are (although they are learning fast) about cancer.

It seemed to me that there were different ways in which we could look at the data upon which the Government made its decisions. Yet, we were committed – or being committed, depending on your personal perspective on the lockdown restrictions – based on just one interpretation of that data. I am not saying those conclusions reached by no doubt well-meaning scientists were wrong. That is not my field of expertise. But similarities between attempts to control Covid 19 and efforts to manage cancer suggested themselves strongly. We rightly trust our oncologists. We should do that. They are the experts. But, maybe, they are not always right. There could be other actions we, as sufferers from cancer, might want to explore.

This book is, in the main, about how I reached my own conclusions about my cancer; the evidence I gathered – not all of it scientific; the research I did. The route I chose to follow.

I say again, this book does not offer a cure for cancer. Any more than it offers the key to becoming a successful international lawyer. Everybody is different; everybody's cancer is unique to them. Everybody's cure could be bespoke to them. But this book tells what I did. It worked for me.

Advocate Altaf Hussain, Solicitor of The Courts of England & Wales, multi Law Society award winning International Lawyer, Chairman of Addison Aaron International Lawyers.

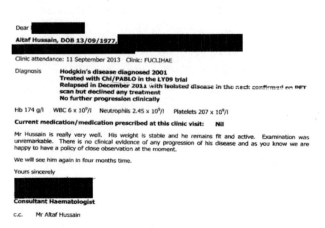

Dear ▮▮▮▮

Altaf Hussain, DOB 13/09/1977, ▮▮▮▮▮▮▮▮▮▮▮

Clinic attendance: 11 September 2013   Clinic: FUCLIHAE

Diagnosis   **Hodgkin's disease diagnosed 2001**
Treated with Chl/PABLO in the LY09 trial
Relapsed in December 2011 with isolated disease in the neck confirmed on PET scan but declined any treatment
No further progression clinically

Hb 174 g/l   WBC 6 x 10⁹/l   Neutrophils 2.45 x 10⁹/l   Platelets 207 x 10⁹/l

Current medication/medication prescribed at this clinic visit: Nil

Mr Hussain is really very well. His weight is stable and he remains fit and active. Examination was unremarkable. There is no clinical evidence of any progression of his disease and as you know we are happy to have a policy of close observation at the moment.

We will see him again in four months time.

Yours sincerely

Consultant Haematologist

c.c.   Mr Altaf Hussain

Copy of the letter at the beginning of the Introduction.

Hostile Witness

The year 2000 seemed such a turning point to so many people. A marker in time which gained almost mystical significance in our lives. I suppose that the much-rumoured Millennium Bug played its part in that.

For younger readers, this was the sudden discovery that the collective weight of mankind's technological brilliance and power, its innovation and originality, might have forgotten to tell computers that the year 2000 existed. The fear spread that, at midnight on December 31st, 1999 (it seems so long ago), every computer in the world would take a collective sigh and think, 'Oh, another year begins. No, actually, another decade. Wow wait a minute, a new century. A new millennium! Help.' Of course those little boxes of programmed thought would make those deductions in far less time than it takes to read their written words, and, a nanosecond later would realise that they didn't actually know what a millennium was, and so would immediately put their clocks back to the year 1900. Since, the theory went, computers were clever enough to realise that they had not been invented in 1900, they would breath another, much happier, collective sigh, and think that they could therefore enjoy a short nap for the next three quarters of a century before the mid-seventies appeared once more, and a few American geeks decided that an upgrade on the typewriter was what the world needed. Again.

Fortunately, or I would be typing this on a black ribbon Remington (look it up, if you don't understand that reference), the bug either had an inbuilt cure or was a little side-show dreamt up by MillenniumMarketing.Com to build anticipation for the upcoming 'big day'. Fortunately, those clever little computers realised that 1999/12/31, 23.59 and 59 seconds was followed by a two, then rather a lot of zeroes.

Like many others, I spent the last night of the twentieth century celebrating away. We had gone down to London, to a house party, about twenty of us. Then over to Tower Bridge, fireworks and screaming 'Happy New Year' to friends and strangers alike. Life was good. I was halfway through a part time course at Birmingham University, studying for my law degree. At the same time, I was working from nine to five as a legal clerk at a commercial law firm in Birmingham, garnering very important experience for the career I had, after a few internal battles and the odd academic disappointment (more about which, later) decided upon. On a Tuesday and Thursday evening, I'd make the short trek across town to the University buildings in Perry Barr for three hours of intensive study. Six o clock to nine o'clock, and then over to Small Heath park for ten. Or, perhaps, over to Paradise Snooker, or a party with friends in the city.

That law firm was Dass Solicitors, 50 Newhall Street. The job was varied, but intense. One moment I might be assisting with the preparation of court bundles, which – as impressive as that sounds – involved standing at the photocopier, running through hundreds of pages of documents. But the next, I could be carrying out legal research for senior lawyers at the firm, providing them with vital background to the case they were preparing. My tea making also came on leaps and bounds during those days, I swear I could have won gold for the best Indian tea in town.

It was a lot of work, but my father had drilled into me from a young age, keep your head down and work hard. Maybe it was later in my early years that the message hit home, but now it had, and I was enjoying the consequences. I also lived a fulfilling and active social life, and plenty of sport on top, but I was young, energetic, and had a clear direction to my life. As I say, life was good. Busy, but good. Very busy, in fact. Perhaps, in the light of what happened next, too busy. I don't know.

The commercial firm with whom I was gaining that much needed experience used to take on a lot of Spanish law students who wanted to experience first-hand an insight into the British system, and I had developed a lot of friends from that sunny part of

Europe. Hence it was that, eight months after the celebrations which marked the turn of the year 2000, I was celebrating another important milestone. This time, it was the marriage of a Spanish friend of ours, Guzman Garcia, who had come from mainland Europe to work with us in the law firm. He had spent six months there, gaining experience. I was in Madrid, with Tony and looking forward to a day out in the sunny city, spending time with friends.

I was in the bathroom, having my morning shave, when I saw it. A small, innocuous looking bump on my neck. I was twenty-two, still barely out of adolescence. Lumps and bumps were a part of life. Anyway, I was in Spain. Clearly, I had been bitten by a mosquito, or some other local insect, although the bump did not itch or hurt like a mosquito bite normally would. I decided next that I must have been stung by a bee in my sleep and slept through the pain. I can't stress enough here that to give four lines to the discovery of that small bump is five lines too many. Like most of us would, I gave it a push and a poke, thought, 'that's a bit odd,' and intended to get on with my day. I was only due to remain in Spain for five days, and I wanted to make the most of every minute. But that morning, I did feel under the weather. I had absolutely no intention of giving anything more than a passing nod to a strange lump on the side of my neck. Probably, thinking back, my main concern was that it might turn into an unsightly spot or boil. Or, perhaps even, an abscess. But I gave no more consideration to the lump than the world's computers had to the mysterious but ultimately harmless non-event that was the Millennium Bug. Yet the feeling of not being quite right persisted, and in the end, I decided that it would be wrong to risk spoiling Guzman's wedding by being taken ill. I decided to stay in my hotel room and rest. It was a shame, having travelled so far, to miss my friend's big day, but my other mates who had travelled with me, Tony, Uncle Charlie (who was nobody's uncle) and Rick, were still able to go. I felt sure that I was making the right decision.

Even back then I loved Spain, and I still do today. I have travelled there a lot, visiting most of the main attractions and travelling at least once to all of its major islands. In fact, I love the whole of mainland Europe. A year before this lump appeared, I had completed a back-packing trip travelling all over Spain, Italy and France. Now, I was going to make the most of the short holiday I had. That was the last consideration I gave to the small blemish on the side of my neck.

Despite missing the wedding, I had a good time in Spain that September. My friends were great company, Tony was a trainee solicitor, Rick worked there as well. Uncle Charlie was neither a relation to any of us, nor older than us either. Sometime, in the deep, distant past, he had acquired the sobriquet which seemed to move him a generation back from his laddish peers, and it had stuck. We were good mates, fun loving and

19

responsible. Usually. Mostly. We looked the part as well, enjoying the sun wearing jeans with a white t shirt and thin designer shirt on top of that. We'd eat paella and seek out the gatherings and parties. We met up with a couple of other friends from when they too had travelled to England to gain experience at the firm. My memory of Spain that late summer is of sun and olives, olive oil and more sun. The country has a deep history, and not always a good one. In the middle ages, it was ruled by Muslims, and prejudice remains in outposts towards my religion. I remember one night we planned to go to a specific club, but Maria and Ana said that, because I was a Muslim, they would make it difficult for us to get in. Despite the underlying racism, I loved the country back then, and still do today.

After the last few days in Spain, I returned to Birmingham intent on studying for the penultimate year of my law degree. It is an often-overused cliché that the world is a person's oyster. While it doesn't stop the phrase being a cliché, for me back in the formative months of the new century, that really was the case. As we will see in the next chapter, I had had a happy upbringing, but not always an easy one. Brought into England from my native Bangladesh at the age of five, with no language and living in a crowded flat in London, I had moved to Small Heath in Birmingham when still a young boy. Like many immigrants, and non-immigrants alike, I had been subject to bullying from time to time, and that (plus a personality that likes to see the funny side of everything) had turned me into the class clown. While such a persona helps to keep one popular, it is not always a best fit for a successful set of school days. But now, having grown up, I really could see a bright and cheery future as a well-paid, successful professional in a career I was growing to find ever more interesting, ever more challenging and ever more fulfilling.

But by the next month, I was beginning to have doubts that the lump on my neck might be quite as innocent as I had first thought. Not only was it not going away, but it was getting bigger. I started to fixate about it, checking it at first daily, then soon much more regularly than that. I tried to think back to anything that might have been the cause of this icon of my anxiety. Had I nicked myself shaving, and allowed the spot to become infected? Had a post-teenage zit appeared, and become septic?

Dr Google was still in training, and it would be a while before he became the world's worst medic – managing to evoke huge worry in his ready supply of patients and getting his diagnosis wrong with alarming regularity. Still, I asked myself what kind of infections, viruses and diseases might be behind this growing facial disfigurement.

Men are notoriously bad at taking problems with their body seriously. Actually, that is probably a little unfair. What they do with lumps and bumps, or variances in their internal clocks, is worry about them, imagine all sorts of fatal consequences for their discomfort, or the change in their toilet habits, or the rash or growth under their skin...and then do nothing about it. I was like that in some manners, but not others. I suppose, in a way, it is too my credit that I left the lump for only a month to six weeks before seeking medical advice.

So, in October 2000, I made an appointment to see my GP. He examined the lump, asked all the usual questions: 'When did it appear?', 'Did it cause discomfort?', 'Did I have any ideas from where it might have originated?'

There was a lot of 'umming' and 'aahing' in the usual of manner of GPs faced with something they cannot easily explain. Then, he followed the line of least resistance employed by so many of his colleagues over the years. He prescribed a course of anti-biotics and told me to 'come back if it doesn't get any better.'

I do not blame my GP. I left his surgery mildly relieved and expecting to see a gradual diminishing of the problem before it finally disappeared. Another slight error in programming of this astonishing mixture of water and organs we call the human body which had allowed a few unwanted microbes to enter, reproduce, and cause me a small problem. An invasion easily repulsed with a few capsules of killer chemicals prescribed by my doctor. I was twenty-two years old, fit, healthy, sports playing and had no record of medical problems. How could he know that this lump was anything but a minor inconvenience easily rectified?

So, I continued with life, waiting for the lump to go away. Except, it didn't. It got bigger. And now it stopped being a benign annoyance on my surface features. By November, just two months since I had first seen the protuberance make its unwelcome appearance, I was beginning to display other symptoms. Very disturbing ones. They started with sudden, excruciating earaches. This painful discomfort is intrusive at the best of times, but these examples were especially severe. As the month progressed, they became ever harsher and ever more regular. For the first time, I started to become seriously worried. I really was not the sort of person to get ill; like many of my age at the time, I felt I was invincible. I was playing football regularly and kept up my other sports as well. I ran and worked out at the gym. Illness was the rarest and most unwelcome of visitors to my home; now it was as though he had not only come to dinner but had refused to leave and had taken up noisy and intrusive residence in the spare room. More than this, the visiting nuisance was spreading out through the entire house. Such was his over-riding presence, that even when he occasionally went out on his own, his odorous aura remained behind, chipping away in the corner of my mind.

The earaches got worse. It is hard to describe the pain. It throbbed in waves of agony, absorbing all of my attention, inducing nausea through its severity. The pain was so intense that I became light-headed with it, unable to concentrate on anything. I felt increasingly weak and my appetite went. I began to lose weight and even more alarmingly, I would get short of breath at the slightest exercise. I was getting weaker. My life was changing.

I followed my doctor's advice and returned to the surgery. This time, the decision was that a deeper examination was required. I was sent to the hospital just before Christmas in 2000, to have a biopsy on the lump. My parents took me to the Heartlands Hospital in Birmingham. Their son sat in the car, nervous and anxious. I have never been one to be scared, but I was a little that day. I guess it is the things we cannot handle which are sent to test us. I was given a sedative before the biopsy and remember waking up with a mouth so dry that I craved something sweet and cold. I was also devastatingly hungry, but I could not move my neck, and was bandaged up. I remember a sense of surprise when my mates Subs and Ash along with a few others, turned up at the hospital with a sandwich and a bottle of juice. That juice was the best I have ever tasted, because my mouth was so dry. I can never forget the sweet sensation of that drink flowing into my throat, cleansing my mouth.

I still have the scar from the biopsy today. A small mark on the left-hand side of my neck. Every time I have a shave it is there to remind me of the pain, the dryness in my mouth. I suppose it was the intervention of Christmas and New Year which meant I had to spend a longer than normal nervous time awaiting the result. My worries were mostly for my parents and my sisters; I found, with the confidence of youth, that I was just hoping for the best. It was as though I could not quite rationalise the magnitude of what I was being tested for. My weight was starting to drop, but I still did not relate that to the disease that was already churning up the insides of my body.

The diagnosis which came back was something that I had refused to allow to even cross my mind. My lump was a symptom of Hodgkin's Lymphoma. I had cancer.

Learning the Law

Is there a creature more majestic than the Bengal Tiger? Ten feet long, weighing more than three times that of the average human, it is also intelligent. Its brain is the size of that of a chimpanzee, and its short-term memory would be considered long term in a human, being thirty times as extensive as that of man. This beautiful beast is famed for its power and courage; respected and also feared among the peoples and prey who share its territory. Its stripes are skin deep, but its strength and bravery go much further than this, right to the heart of the creature. Although it once roamed over much of south Asia, today its numbers are concentrated in parts of India, and they are dwindling to such an extent that the Bengal tiger faces the threat of extinction.

Such an outcome would be an irredeemable, inexcusable loss to the planet. And, especially, to the people of Bangladesh, where the Bengal tiger is the nation's national animal, worshipped among some of the indigenous people, such as the Warli. In Bangladesh, the beast is found in the enormous forest of the Sundarbans, in the south of the country around the Bay of Bengal. The forest is a UNESCO World Heritage site and recognised as one of the natural wonders of the world. The Sundarbans contains networks of marine streams which flow between mud shores and through mangrove forests filled with exotic birds, reptiles, snakes and, sadly, rarest of them all, the tiger.

But if the great beast is an endangered species, back in 1977 the world too was undergoing troubled times. It was the year of the great New York blackout, when the city lost power for more than a day – good news for the looters, bad for everybody else. It marked, astonishingly, the final execution by guillotine in France, before the country decided to move its judicial system out of the seventeenth century and into the 1970s. In further human rights violations, South Africa was plunged into one of its worst years of apartheid atrocities; the year also saw the death, in police custody, of journalist Steve Biko.

It was a bad year for the aviation industry, with one of the biggest air disasters of all time occurring when five hundred and eighty-three people died following the collision of two jumbo jets on a runway in the Canary Islands. Later in the year a flight from Paris to Tokyo was hijacked by the Japanese Red Army, with a hundred and fifty-six people on board. It had stopped in Bombay, but on the final leg of its journey to Japan was forced to fly to Bangladesh, and land in Dhaka. The Japanese government's decision to give in to the terrorists' demand caused anxiety in the West but saved the lives of the hostages. 1977 was also the year that Elvis Presley died, and I was born. For the first time ever, of the fraction short of seventy-five million people who inhabited Bangladesh in that year (according to the inestimably reliable source that is Wikipedia), one was me. And that statistic would remain so, at least for the next five years.

Bangladesh in the mid to late seventies was an uncertain place. The newly formed nation had gained independence from Pakistan only six years previously, and its recently elected President, Ziaur Rahman, faced a number of attempts to overthrow his fledgling Government. To be fair, political unrest didn't mean a lot to the baby in arms that was me. Eating, sleeping, defecating and being hugged accounted for much of my time, and I wasn't even interested to note that this was the year that Bangladesh became an associate member of the International Cricket Council, although, to be fair, I would have been a lot more interested in this sporting detail had it happened a few years later.

In fact, I hold few memories of Bangladesh, because when I was only shortly out of nappies, I followed older generations of my family and emigrated to Britain, living in a small flat in a relatively run down part of London. Still, I was fortunate to spend my first five years in the mystical nation that is Bangladesh. I was born in a small village called Uthor Akakazna, in Beani Bazar, Sylhet, a medium sized city in a region famed for tea growing and natural resources such as gas and oil. Like so many other parts of the former Indian sub-continent, its history is pock-marked by the rule of both the Mughal Empire of the seventeenth and eighteenth centuries, and following the fall of that, the colonial reign of the British Empire. This was initially under the control of the British East India Company, who based themselves in the Bengal before spreading out over the remainder of the sub-continent. Later, with that political entity disbanded, having committed one atrocity too many, the British army, under the rule of Parliament and Victoria, took over. Nevertheless, Sylhet retains some inspiring and important architecture. It is famed for its Sufi shrines, including the beautiful and intricate tomb and mosque of Hazrat Shaha Jalal, a fourteenth century saint. The site is now a destination for pilgrims and is situated near the Dargah Gate. Sylhet can lay claim to another remarkable boast, albeit one which is inevitably held by one part of any nation. It is the region from which most people emigrate to the west. In Britain, that destination is often the central London region of Tower Hamlets, although when I moved to the country's capital in the early 1980s it was a little to the south and across the Thames from this infamous borough. Our destination being the evocatively named Elephant and Castle, best known for appearing as the final stop on some south travelling tube trains on the Northern line. (With apologies, of course, to Morden.)

My great grandad Mokodor Ali was the first of our family to head west to Europe. He had been an important member of his community in Bangladesh, a leader and an advocate in our village who spent many of his waking hours involved in settling land disputes. He worked for a shipping company and arrived in England in the early 1960s. What a strange and disturbing place he must have found. A country which relied on workers from afar, both the east and the west, yet remained filled with the lingering spores of a racist empire.

Nevertheless, my grandfather, Motosin Ali, and my father, Moynul Hoque (Shamsul), soon too made the decision to seek out new horizons in Europe and joined their own father/grandfather in London. Life was hard for these early immigrants, and not just in the way they could be regarded by the native population. Remember, these were the days of television comedy shows which based their entire supposed humour around the mocking of racial stereotypes – 'It Ain't Half Hot, Mum,' (about an army concert party based somewhere in India, towards the end of the second world war, in which jokes centred around the fact that the tough sergeant major used the word 'poof' a lot, about his recruits, and the one significant Indian character was played by a white British actor wearing black face who could do a neck wobble.' 'Mind your language' was another, which at least had the good grace to deride any nationality which was not British, rather than just black ones, and 'Love thy Neighbour' where we laughed so hard at hearing words such as 'Sambo' and 'Honky' that the walls shook. Or not.

But my senior generations also worked unbelievably hard for their cramped rooms in London and Birmingham. I remember my grandfather telling me that he was employed in numerous factories, including the BSA (Birmingham Small Arms), a gunmakers, at one time, was the biggest manufacturer of weaponry in Europe. My dad, too, slogged away at building a life for himself. He had left school at fourteen, working in restaurants in London.

As was the norm in those days, although he was living in England dad would travel back each year to Bangladesh. Under the arranged marriage system, a few potential brides were sorted for him, and he chose my mum, Husneara Begum. They were married in 1976. He was in London when I was born on September 13th of the following year.

By the time I arrived in London, along with my mother, to live with my father's aunt in that Elephant and Castle flat, he had already established his own business. He and his cousin ran a grocery company on the Wandsworth Road, in SW8 of London. This is Vauxhall, close to the Oval cricket ground and a part of the larger borough of Lambeth. One of my earliest memories is of seeing my father driving off to work in his red van. Sometimes we would squeeze into the back, maybe six of us, to travel to see relatives. It was hot, steamy but, to a small child, great fun. The flat in which we lived, cramped, at least could boast a balcony, and I would move onto it whenever I could, and play with toy aeroplanes while the real thing flew overhead, descending on its flightpath to land at Heathrow.

Of course, it didn't mean a huge amount to the barely more than an infant me, but in some ways I had left the political uncertainties of Bangladesh behind (although, in rural Beani Bazar we were in many ways sheltered from them) for a different kind of unrest in Britain. In 1982, the Prime Minister, Margaret Thatcher, secured her place in posterity by sending a battle fleet to other side of the world to liberate a group of small, wind beaten islands from Argentinian control. The Falklands. With two opposing nations each claiming ownership of these small pieces of rock, and with each of their leaders, Galtieri (who ran the Argentinian junta) and the aforementioned Thatcher, seeking to use the conflict to further their own political aims, both politically and internationally, Britain was a country driven by a surge of patriotic zeal. That made the nation a tough place for one culturally and racially different, who couldn't speak the language and was bamboozled by the weird conventions of primary school.

Maybe that was a part of the reason my school days are ones that, by and large, I look back upon with a mixture of a sense of missed opportunity and, incongruously, disappointed affection. Or perhaps I was just a naughty boy, some of the time at least. Whatever, I was constantly in trouble in school. Never major, exclusion threatening, trouble, but instructions to 'concentrate', 'get on' and 'stop disturbing others'. Occasionally, I fell victim to bullying but such was my sense of justice, I could never bow down before a bigger foe. That cost me a few beatings.

Yet in many ways I enjoyed a great time. I was the class clown, the one who was constantly fooling around and sending my teachers grey, or greyer than they already were. Like so many before and after me, I reflect back now and think about how much more I could have achieved had I been inclined to work consistently, get my head down and do my best. And although I make no excuses about my lack of academic (or behavioural, to be fair) fortitude, from an adult perspective I do see the culture of my adopted country back in those days of the eighties as contributing to the way I viewed life. All children are highly susceptible to influences around them, and during that time the culture of self above community, of almost jingoistic fervour, of money ruling over everything, was immensely strong. Remember, these were the days of 'Loadsamoney', of Poll Tax riots, of extremes of football hooliganism that shook the country, and made Saturday afternoons no go times in many town centres.

Life as an only child ended shortly after I arrived in England. The following year my first of four sisters came along. Forhana Begum was born in London, in the small flat.   It soon became apparent that living with a great Aunt in a tiny London apartment was not going to be sustainable. We moved to Birmingham, taking a maisonette close to the Blues (Birmingham City) football ground. It was there, in 1984, that my second sister was born. Sofrana Begum. Another sibling, and another sister, arrived in 1990, by which time we had moved to our home in Small Heath, on Tennyson Road. Shabina Begum and the rest of us were eventually joined by my youngest sister, Salina Begum, who was born in 1995, by which time I was eighteen.

Growing up as an older brother made me incredibly protective of my sisters. I remember, for example, although I cannot recall why, feeling that I was their guardian against bees. I recall at the age of nine seeing a bumble bee (which are, of course, the most benign of stinging beasts, despite their large appearance) on our window sill, and attacking it with a teddy bear to save my sister from being stung. Which, of course, would not have happened had I simply left the poor creature alone. Unfortunately, both myself and the teddy bear paid a price, the bee defending itself by stinging me (fatally, no doubt, for the insect itself) and the teddy bear sacrificing an eye as it headbutted the window sill in an attempt to repel the invader. Bees ran strongly in my role as defender of my sisters. I was around twelve when Forhana and Sofrana were attacked by a swarm of the buzzing beasts on the way to the mosque. Bravely, I stepped in, getting stung for my troubles once more.

I still am, in a way, protective of my siblings even today. Yet we enjoy a terrific relationship. I suppose that in many circumstances being an older brother was the area in which I did show responsibility, in a childish but well-meaning manner, as a boy.

But to return to our move from that London flat, we headed north and the spot my parents chose was in Birmingham, firstly into the maisonette in which Sofrana was born which sat just two minutes from St Andrew's, the Birmingham City football stadium, and then to another part of Small Heath. These days, the area is probably best known for being the stamping ground of the Peaky Blinders, a criminal gang glorified in the eponymous BBC series. Culturally, Small Heath was more of a home from home for us, at least compared to the Elephant and Castle. With over half of its population of Pakistani descent at the time, and more than a quarter from other southern Asian nations, we settled easily for the most part.

However, there were moments of tension. In fact, there was quite a lot of violence, and racism from Pakistani and Afghan boys. But, as I have said, whilst I did not instigate fights, I also did not back down from them. In the end, I began to emerge as a leader among the local kids, and that helped me to establish some wide friendships across the community.

My dad had sold his grocery shop in London, and had joined his brother, Soyful, to work in the Birmingham restaurant trade. It was with Soyful, along with his wife and daughter, that the five of us (myself, mum, dad, Forhana and Sofrana) had lived with on first arriving in Birmingham, in that small three bedroomed maisonette. To say it was cramped is an understatement. I used to make the fifteen-minute walk to Regent's Park Primary school on my own, even from the age of seven. I remember, one day, a dreadful wind blew up and it was strong enough to knock me over. I was scared but going to school on my own helped me to grow up. Years later on her discovery, mum said to me: 'If I knew your school was that far, I'd never have let you walk there on your own.'

I didn't see much of dad in those early years in Birmingham, as he was committed to working double shifts at the restaurant. It was that work ethic which later allowed him, along with his brother, to set up his own place. Peppers' Restaurant, in Studley, Warwickshire.

But even by primary school, sport was driving my life. I was made captain of the school football team and represented Regent's Park in the 100m sprint. In fact, I was usually captain of any football team in which I played. I did have, right from a young age, good leadership skills. My football was pretty good back then. I started out as a pacy winger, then moved to midfield as I got older. I finished my footballing days as a striker; less need to run around then! As a boy, growing up during the days of Liverpool's dominance in the league, I supported them along with Birmingham City. The Blues were my local club of course, and for a time I lived by the ground. But I found the stress of being a fan took away the joy of watching games. I enjoyed the 2019/20 Liverpool team finally winning the Premier League, but not in the way I would have done twenty five years ago.

In those youthful days, I used to build up my speed by racing against the local buses as they chugged down the main road. I can't imagine what the locals made of a small boy charging at full pelt down the high road, apparently chasing a number 60 bus, or whichever double decker was making its way at that moment, then on the rare occasions he actually caught it up, refusing to board. Still, it all made sense to me.

Not though, that this helped me to behave myself in school. Firstly, the teachers at Regents Park School, then later at Small Heath School, the local secondary, were subject to the laughs, jokes and (I have to admit) the more than occasional fights which a bright, sporty but somewhat lazy pupil got himself into. I have always had a finely attuned sense of justice; I suppose that in part accounts for the career which I ultimately decided to pursue. Perhaps it was a good thing, perhaps it wasn't but I even got into a fight on my very first day of secondary school. I was playing football with a small group of friends, when a gang tried to take our ball. They obviously thought that we would be easy meat. Furious, I launched an offensive which not only saw us retain our football, but also earned me the reputation as the 'hardest boy in the year.' That's important, when you are eleven. No doubt, though, on the other side it helped to furnish in me an undeserved reputation with some of the teachers. Yet, for all that, I must have been seen as a likeable enigma to those hard-pressed staff. I was definitely popular with them, although I understand now that I was also probably frustrating to teach.

On another occasion, I was on the receiving end of an undeserved attack. I was in small heath park, aged around thirteen, when a group of about ten to fifteen Pakistani rebels surrounded me. They asked if I was a Bengali, and when I stated that I was, they jumped me, carrying out a bizarre attack based presumably on the fact that Bangladesh had, many years before, gained independence from their own homeland. It was weird, to be attacked for a cause which was centred on lands thousands of miles away, and from a couple of decades before. I can honestly say that I never started a fight, but my sense of right and wrong was highly defined, if perhaps naïve in its youthfulness, and therefore I was prepared to defend myself, my beliefs and the rights of others. This time, though, as hard as I fought, I still ended up with a beating, and a number of painful bruises.

I was always brave. I think it was my dad's uncle, Azmol Ali, who helped me to develop my courage. He lived in Portsmouth before moving to Birmingham. I went to stay with him and his wife, Bina, in 1987 when I was ten. Although they were younger than me, my uncle and aunt were there, Azmal's children, Shahed who was seven, and his sister, Shume, who was four. I had a great summer. I would ride around on Shahed's Raleigh bike, and was always getting into fights over it. Older kids would pull me by my ears, but I always held onto that bike. I went to the seaside, playing on the tanks and the RAF fighter jets, and had great times on Portsmouth beach.

Once Shahed and I took Shume out with us but left her on the roof of the seventeenth floor of the block of flats. It was terrible, anything could have happened to her. Azmol was so angry. Uncle Shahed and I remain friends, sharing more than just an uncle to nephew relationship, to this day, unless of course we are playing tennis.

It was around the time that I spent the summer in Portsmouth that I took up karate. Dad is a huge Bruce Lee fan and has all the films. On his day off from his work at the restaurant we would sit down together and watch a Jacki Chan movie. It was quite traditional at home. Mum was the housewife, and she never really gained a good grasp of English. My karate classes were in Digbeth, near the city centre, and I would catch a bus there. It was fine when the nights were light, but as Autumn arrived and the dark set in earlier and earlier, I used to be fearful alone on the bus. I was only ten, and winter was a scary time. I think, though, that being encouraged to grow up quickly, and take responsibility for myself, helped me a lot. It was those experiences as a youngster which helped me become confident and brave as I got older.

When I was twelve, I stopped going to karate and took up kung fu. The Master used to say that I needed discipline and would beat me. Perhaps I was a little cocky. One day he, along with a senior student, picked me up and ripped my legs apart. That was when I learned to do the splits (something I still do today. I kept up my kung fu for a number of years, and later when I was in my twenties, I tried out a few other martial arts. They have always fascinated me, the combination of strict discipline and controlled aggression. I still have a punch bag in my garage, where I can hammer out the stresses of a difficult day at the office.

It was just before I took up karate, when I was in the latter stages of primary school, that we moved out of the cramped maisonette and into our new house in Tennyson Road. This is a mixed street, next to small heath park, with some large properties, but also some smaller ones tucked together.

Yet in Birmingham, when I was still a boy, despite my reputation as a 'hard man' I wasn't at all, really. I was into fashion – later I got a leather Guns and Roses biker's jacket which I wore proudly and casually – I even (when I was old enough to grow them) bore a pair of Elvis Presley style sideburns. The nineties have much to answer for, in terms of fashion. Or, perhaps, it is just me. That Mr Cool Guy image threatened to take a bit of a beating when I was fifteen and spent two weeks staying in a French convent with nuns. We lived off bread, soup and cheese. The purpose of the trip was for work experience, and I spent the fortnight working in a chemist's near Paris. It was here, on my first trip away from family, that I tasted my first cigarette. *Oh bonjour!*

To be fair, and honest, I was a bit of a cocky kid growing up. One day I was playing football in the park and rode home – as was usually the case – on my bike.

'Is that yours?' a man asked once, suspiciously.

'Course it is,' came my assured reply.

The next thing I knew I had been grabbed from the bike and received a kick in the stomach. The man had mistaken my confidence for cheekiness and had handed out his own response to that.

Once, I experienced another brush with violence, one which could have had far more serious consequences. I had got into fights over the 'tax' demanded by thugs from the streets surrounding my school. Basically, a gang would demand money to stop them from beating us up. I was never going to pay, even it meant having to fight to make my point. My dad worked hard for what we had and wasn't intending to hand any cash over to any Tom, Dick or Hassan. Once, before school, I was approached by two English boys who demanded their 'tax'. When I refused to pay, they produced a butcher's knife and began to threaten me with it. Unfortunately for them, I stood up to them and like most bullies, they soon backed off. I ended up chasing them away.

In fact, it was my love of sports, which continues to this day, was probably my saving grace at school. That, and the fact that I would fight for people if (I believed) the circumstances so dictated, made me popular with my peers both in school and in the wider community. Sport also motivated me in my academic studies. It was for this subject that I found the motivation to get up in the mornings and get into school for an 8.00am start, completing extra study in anatomy and physiology for my Physical Education GCSE, which I took as an additional subject. I would also take part in numerous sports – athletics, football, cricket, squash, badminton, swimming. I was captain of the school football team and represented them at cricket as well. If only, I reflect from afar, I had put as much effort into my academic studies.

An incident which sticks out in my mind and demonstrates how much I must have frustrated my teachers, involved my GCSE coursework for science. By now, I did have an ambition – to become a doctor, more about which later – but regarded it in that bizarre way typical of teenagers, and especially boys. On the one hand, I was passionate about the subject. I had become fascinated by the stories my mother told of her brother, Bodrul, my uncle, who had so wanted to study medicine but had been unable to complete his courses because his father could not afford it. I was also studying the development of medicine as a part of my History work – learning about Hippocrates, William Harvey, Galen and other leaders in the field. I was quite determined that I would become the family's representative in the world of medicine.

Yet I was a teenage boy. The passion was there, the motivation and organisation needed to realise such ambition was not. I managed to miss the deadline for handing in my science coursework, and my teacher was so frustrated that he tore it up in front of me when I eventually presented it a day late. Seeing a promising student, but one who frequently behaved like a fool, throwing away his future was just too much for him. As for me, I was terrified; distraught by the twin fears that I had blown away my own dreams, and also that my family would be informed of this. I still managed to pass the exam, but the double C grade ruled out science for A levels, necessary requirements for a career in medicine in those days. Instead, I decided on law as the next best aspiration for my career as I had gained a grade A in English in year 10. I would, though, need to settle down and do some work.

I suppose, on reflection, failed ambitions in medicines have not worked out too badly for the family. While my own career as a lawyer has enabled me to become a partner in my own firm, my uncle Bodrul has done pretty well as well. He eventually emigrated to the US and is now a very successful businessman in New York.

I was lucky in that my brain is suited to the British exam system. Even though I never worked as hard as I should, and could, I did well enough in my GCSEs to win a place in the sixth form of one of Birmingham's, and the country's, leading state schools. King Edward's Camp Hill. The school had been sited at Camp Hill, near the City Centre, when it was founded in 1883. But its popularity meant that it outgrew its original site. It took up the campus it still holds, next to its sister school in King's Heath. (King Edward VI Camp Hill School for Boys is its official title and tells us all we need to know). It was, and remains, selective, and I should have been keen to make the most of my time there. I did, in some ways.

Unfortunately, though, not in academic ones, and my dream of going to Cambridge or Oxford was drifting away. The grammar school culture of getting one's head down, following the rules and the glory of the academic did not sit well with the sixteen-year-old me. I was rebellious, lazy and, I have to say, probably at my worst in terms of becoming an archetypal teenage dosser. Once in King Edward's, I quickly teamed up with a friend from primary school, Feraz Rauf. We spent far too much time looking good, and having fun to commit to study. Town became our regular hangout joint, fitted tight tops, flexing our triceps. I like to consider myself a 'chiller.'

Birmingham has a strong rock scene, and not just for spawning Ozzie Osbourne. Music thrilled me. I liked to look cool, with my Elvis sideburns and Beverley Hills 90210 fashion sense. I wore flared bootcut jeans and enjoyed an eclectic love of music. Everything from Buddy Holly, to the Beatles, to Bon Jovi to Guns'n'Roses. Despite my campaign to become Small Heath's own fashion guru, I did manage to keep up my sport, playing for the school football team, and was selected for the quiz team as well, but as for working for my A levels in English, History and Economics? Not a chance. Those exams seemed too far away to matter, and when they suddenly loomed up, knocking at my front door, it was already too late to catch up missed study. I really had blown it; I was an able student and had even taken English GCSE a year early, gaining an A grade despite completing the course in advance of normal time, but this time I had left it too late.

Yet at eighteen failing my A levels seemed almost a mark of achievement, at least, that is what I told myself, and I refused to remain at King Edward's to complete my retakes. Instead, I enrolled at a sixth form college closer to the city centre. Matthew Boulton College had a reputation, back then, as a place for hard nuts. I might have been a 'bad boy' by King Edward's standards, but not here. I met all sorts of characters like 'BIG Nav,' Mr Razak, who went onto become a chartered surveyor. Back then we would go to his house in Alum Rock, do our homework, pump our biceps, look in the mirror and eat jacket potatoes.

I dressed the part, developed a suitably aggressive, disinterested manner and, with still less work than I should have employed, managed to finally pass my exams. I was ready to make my way in the world.

It was 1998, and the promise of new starts was on the horizon. My sister, Sofrana, saw an advert in the paper which said a law firm in the city centre was seeking an office junior. I applied for the job, and Sally Ann Hall gave me my break. The firm also sponsored me to undertake a part time law degree over four years in the evening at Birmingham City University. It was a great opportunity, maybe even one I didn't deserve, given my previously laid-back approach to academia.

But I had grown up and seized the chance to make something of my life.

To help me with that, I had already enjoyed two significant experiences which had pointed me in the direction I wanted to follow. Certainly, my academic successes as a school boy were much less than they might have been, but much more than they would have been had I not, firstly at the age of ten and then when I was fifteen, enjoyed lengthy trips to Bangladesh.

My mother and father took me there in 1987 and we stayed for around six months. It was a wonderful time for the class clown, who (on reflection) might not have been as happy as he thought at his primary school. My parents ensured, though, that my education did not suffer during the extended visit. They enrolled me in the local village school, and I also remember the pleasure of just riding my bicycle around the village, so different from the packed houses and streets full of angry cars in Small Heath. When we travelled to see my mother's family, in Kakordi, Beani Bazar in Sylhet, we travelled by boat cruising through overflowing canals and rivers.

Looking back, it seems quite a dangerous and daunting undertaking; at the time it was just huge fun. When I was there, in Kakordi, I would spend my days canoeing with my cousin, Sadat Hoque, paddling through the flooded fields. Sadat died of cancer in 2002. Such a waste of a life and a future. He passed shortly after I pushed my own first bout into long term remission. Sport dominated that half a year break. I played badminton, volleyball, football and would go fishing.

As I have said, I remember almost nothing from my first few years in Bangladesh, but this visit gave me perspective on my life. It helped me, in a small way, to grow up.

I went back again in 1992. With GCSEs on the horizon, this time I went just for the summer holidays, accompanying my uncle, and stayed for about six weeks. Now I was old enough for the experience to be life changing. I returned to Birmingham with newfound determination. It was during this time that I settled on my chosen (but unrequited) career in medicine and committed myself to extra studies before school. Sadly, of course, that passion did not last, and I went back to my old ways. But it had given me an insight into an alternative path for my life, and I am grateful for that.

I'm going to finish this chapter with a mention of my other grandfather, the one from my mother's side, Mahmood Ali. My first proper memories of him are from when I visited Bangladesh with my parents in 1987. I recall a very funny man, who made a big impression on me. He gave me a small, passport sized photograph of himself, and told me to keep it in my pocket, so that he would be with me, and I would be reminded of him. In many ways this was a lesson about the heartache that is caused when your family lives on the other side of the world and you cannot often get to see them. It was a cause of immense pleasure to me that he managed to attend my wedding before he passed away. I carried that photograph of Mahmood Ali in my pocket for a very, very long time.

Maybe the 'hardest boy in the year' had a softer side after all.

Case to Answer

I suppose, looking back later from afar, I did fit some of the risk factors for Hodgkin's Lymphoma. It is a disease that hits men more often than women, and is rare in the cancer world in that it targets the young, with those aged between fifteen and thirty most at risk of the disease, although it comes back to haunt much older people as well. Many of the symptoms from which I suffered in those early days were also conditions which those with the illness often display. Particularly, the painless swelling of lymph nodes – for me, that was the lump in my neck.

The tiredness from which I suffered back in those days late in the year 2000 was also a known warning sign (although, of course, it is also an indicator of many other conditions, including simply not getting enough sleep, something to which the young frequently regularly expose themselves. I certainly was guilty of that). The difficulty I had sleeping, my weight loss and perhaps even the extreme earaches were also indicators that the disease might be present. Other symptoms of the disease include fevers, particularly severe night drenches, and severe itching. An adverse reaction towards alcohol is often experienced, with severe pain in the lymph nodes after having a drink.

Hodgkin's Lymphoma – it used to be known as Hodgkin's disease – it is a cancer that develops in the lymphatic system. As is often the case with cancers, the disease can present itself in many subtly different ways, which is a part of what can make it hard to treat. However, fundamentally a genetic mutation develops in one of the lymph cells – called lymphocytes – and reproduces. Quite quickly, a number of overgrown lymphocytes will gather in a sufferer's lymphatic system. These large and abnormal parasites quickly overwhelm healthy cells, and the symptoms explained above appear. What actually triggers the disease is something doctors are still struggling to discover. As is why it is a disease which disproportionately affects the young, and especially young men. There seems to be a connection to family history, which suggests the potential for there to be some genetic factors behind the likelihood of a person getting the disease. To the best of my knowledge, however, there is no trace of the disease among my predecessors.

Back in the 1970s, Hodgkin's Lymphoma was a serious killer, with nearly half of victims dying within five years. That figure has reduced over time as treatments improve. However, the death rate among men is still high, and was higher still back at the turn of the century when the condition was diagnosed in me.

It was in January of 2001 that I was given the difficult news. I had gone to the hospital and was taken into a small room by a nurse. I recall the room as being dark, poorly lit. Whether that is because of the associations I have with that chamber, or whether it really was dimly lit, I could not say for sure. A cancer nurse told me that I had the disease. She talked through my chemotherapy options, but I was not really able to take it all in. I hope that these days, hospitals are more skilled at giving this kind of news. I am sure that they are. At that moment, my world had collapsed. My hopes, my dreams, my aspirations seemed shattered. I was twenty-three years old. How could this have happened to me? Why was I there, in that room, with that well-meaning nurse?

I was given the choice of two types of chemotherapy. How could I, at my age and with my experience, make that kind of decision? Maybe, if I had worked harder at school and achieved the grades I needed to get into medical school, I would have been in a better position to make a reasoned choice? Maybe. But dealing with somebody else's problems is very different to dealing with our own. I felt like I was playing chess, but against an opponent much stronger than me. If I made the wrong move, this opponent would sweep me aside, checkmating me quickly, and permanently. In the end, opted for treatment through a combination of injections and tablets. This was the ChlVPP/PABLOE option which was part of the LY09 trial. Meaningless. Did the nurse's presentation of the options influence my decision? I have no idea. None at all. I think it was the word 'trial' that tilted my choice. Looking back now, the idea that I chose a trial still freaks me out. This was an unproven route. A gamble. Hit and miss. But I was young. The trial would last six months, and at the end of it they would assess whether I had overcome the cancer inside of me. Six months, twice a week for injections at the hospital, plus a bag full of pills to take at home. Every time I attended the hospital it hit me how young I was, and how old all the other victims seemed to be. Once more, the question of 'Why Me?' filled my brain.

By the time of my diagnosis, my symptoms had become, at times, unmanageable. The earaches were perhaps the worst, the pain so excruciating that I could not think, rationalise, or even operate. They were at times unbearable. I remember one day the pain was so extreme that I had to leave work early. Really, I should have sought help. I recall attempting to walk to the bus stop, just a few minutes away, but after five minutes of agonised movement, I was completely exhausted. I just had no energy at all. It is so hard to describe or imagine for those who have never experienced such fatigue.

I am conscious that my story sounds like hyperbole, a false drama created to move the narrative along. But the exhaustion I felt that winter day just walking to the bus stop was intensely frightening. All the time, my ear throbbed, and nausea swept over me. My head thumped with waves of excruciating pain. I had genuinely never felt such physical distress. And on top of all of this, I could not breathe. The shortness of breath that accompanied my symptoms had become so extreme that day that it actually, physically hurt. Yet, this pain was lost in the maelstrom of agony that ran throughout my body. I was afraid, of course, but somehow that anxiety got lost behind the physical extremes of my discomfort. Every cloud has a silver lining, and all that.

Somehow, I got on the bus. Every jerk of the vehicle sent spasms through my body. Fortunately, as far as I remember, leaving work early meant that I missed most of the worst of the rush hour, and there were seats available. I genuinely wonder if I could have made the lumbering journey back without somewhere to prostrate myself. Yet buses are not the smoothest of vehicles, and the Birmingham traffic, heavy at any time of the day, caused jolting movements, even the whine of the air brakes cutting into my brain like sharp shards of iced glass.

In the end, as you do, somehow, I managed the journey, and from there the short walk to my home. My mother was inside and with maternal concern and motherly understatement asked:

'Are you OK?'

'Yes, of course I'm fine,' I replied, attempting to alleviate the concern spread across her features. I suppose I was attempting, subconsciously, to put on a brave face to hide the fact that I was burning up inside, that the pain was so intense that I could not tell where next breath was coming from. A part of me, deep down, was still refusing to accept the conflict which had taken hold in my body. A battle which, at that stage, was running overwhelmingly in favour of the alien invaders. I was young, fit, healthy and, until very recently, extremely active. Still a part of me reasoned that it would pass. Perhaps that was also behind my denial of my symptoms that day. Yet, you cannot fool your mother, and I have no doubt that she knew how her only son was suffering. That evening, I lay on the sofa and for the first time I realised that I might be dying.

Over the next few weeks, I spent time in and out of hospital, and soon had my own special seat in the surgery waiting room, so frequent a visitor I had become. It was the shortness of breath that was now becoming the most worrying symptom; not being able to breathe really is a very frightening condition. January also marked the time when I began my chemotherapy treatments. I recall going to the hospital with three of my mates, Akbar, Hassan and Akmal. Akbar was a great sportsman, and he and I used to compete at school. We were both county standard in a range of sports. I did not feel county standard as I awaited treatment, though. The poison would be delivered into my body with a mixture of injections and drugs in tablet form. I was given an enormous bag of medicines to take home with me and included among these were anti sickness tablets. But I was a young man, tough, strong (in mind if not, these days, in body) and really felt that I would have no need to take anti sickness drugs. The concept seemed to me, in my early twenties, somehow unworthy. A little weak willed, perhaps. While at an intellectual level I understood that the war inside my body was about to take a new and potentially uncomfortable turn, with my own struggling defences suddenly supplemented by the superweapon of chemotherapy, I genuinely thought the internal collateral damage these drugs would wrought was something against which I could take a deep breath, swallow and stand tall. Youth. It has a lot to answer for. And be proud about.

I took the first load of tablets and thought that I would be OK. For a couple of hours, this belief was reinforced. I was fine. No more than that, admittedly, but coping. Then the nausea started, and the vomiting soon followed. Except, it did not stop. I simply vomited non-stop. My stomach muscles burned; my organs felt scraped raw by the acid which was circulating through them. That dreadful, lightheaded sense of lack of control took hold in my brain and refused to budge for anything. I could not concentrate, my head throbbed. Still, fluid poured until there was nothing left to throw up. But that brought no relief, in fact, in some ways it was worse. The vile discomfort did not cease, nor even pause as it racked through my body, and my fruitless convulsions brought new levels of pain to my tired, agonising muscles.

Dad still worked all hours, and when he arrived home at one o'clock in the morning to find his anxious wife and crippled son there was no doubt what to do. The next of many trips to hospital followed. There I was injected with the anti-nausea drugs I needed all along, and after five nonstop hours, the retching and nausea began to ease. Still, though, the impact on my body remained. It was as though I had been battered by thugs late at night in Birmingham's infamous Bull Ring, beaten to a pulp but with every wound on the inside.

For the next six months I was wrecked by the chemotherapy my body was trying to absorb. I could not work. I could not go to University. At the hospital I would receive painful injections. I remember one day early on in my treatment the sun shining despite the fact that it was the middle of winter. I had received my injection, and also some anti-sickness pills, and decided that I did not feel too bad. I even went to the park, enjoying the chilled air and bright early year sun. I got home, and took the second dose of chemo at about 8.00 pm. Once more, sickness followed, and again I endured perhaps four hours of solid vomiting until yet another one of the frequent hospital visits I endured was enforced, my parents again stepping in to provide the support and security I needed.

But this time, even the hospital could not help. As fast as they pumped the much-needed anti-nausea drugs into me, so I vomited them out. The unequal battle continued for two hours. It was like trying to fill an old bucket with water. As fast as the essential fluid was poured in, so the bucket leaked it out. Except, the bucket that was me had developed a spinning, rotating engine which threw the anti-sickness drugs out with violent force, as though they were the aggressors, evicted like violent drunks in a nightclub by over-zealous bouncers. My body could not recognise, that night, influences sent to calm it, to ease it. It was three a.m. before the determined doctors finally won the day, and the vomiting stopped. I was left like an old, deflated punch bag. Sore and hanging, wanting nothing more than to lie on the ground, alone, and clear of this debilitating disease and the outrageous effects of the treatment intended to send it on its way.

The injections of poison into my body had to be given twice a week. I dreaded those visits to hospital. Often, my friends would accompany me – it was tremendously good, and loyal, of them. But the hospital would not allow them into the ward where I would receive my treatment. There is no getting away from it, these needles hurt. I would feel this chilled, freezing cold ache run up my arm as the chemotherapy was thrust into my body. I suppose that the chemicals had to be kept in a fridge, but they were really painful. It didn't help that I was becoming little more than a bag of skin and bone. Because I was really active and looked after my body through the sports I enjoyed, along with sessions at the gym and so forth, I was never especially heavy, so had no protective layer of flesh to call upon. I was young, as well, and my metabolism would burn calories as fast as I could thrust them in. I threw away around one and a half stones over those first few weeks of chemotherapy. But weight was not all I lost.

I recall on many occasions heading to the hospital, nodding goodbye to friends as I was called into the cancer ward for my injections. As I was about to enter the ward each time I would look into the cancer ward through the window, with its exceptionally sick residents, who all seemed so old and so helpless. The feeling would hit me, 'I shouldn't be here. This is not me. I am too young for this. I am too fit, too healthy. I am not a victim of cancer.'

But I was. Although, I was by now beginning to understand that my attitude towards being such a victim might define my battle with the disease. But those ruminations were still fledgling beings in my mind, and it was the physical indignities that were holding most of my attention.

One day, quite soon after I began taking my course of chemotherapy, I ran my hand through my hair. I cannot recall what prompted this; it is, after all, an everyday action most of us undertake regularly.

Usually, without giving the slightest consideration to it. But this time, the unconscious act stuck in my mind. As I pulled my hand up and out of my hair, I was aware that it did not feel as it should. I looked, and there covering my hand, and onto my arm, were clumps of my hair. Of course, I understood that a by-product of chemotherapy is hair loss. But until it happened it just seemed like one of those distant threats, dangers too far away to (for the most part) be allowed in the forefront of my thinking. Now, suddenly, the reality hit. It was a blow that was almost physical in its intensity. I realised that I would go bald. This might seem a trivial side effect. But it is not. I don't know whether the loss of hair impacts more on the young, I suspect not.

That cancer has no part of you, it is an alien whom you have not invited in. To cause such clear and apparent damage is sickening. I cannot stress this enough.

Over the next few weeks, the threat became a reality. It was not just the hair on my head that began to abandon me, like frightened members of the crew of an endangered ship. Soon, my eyelashes and eyebrows were giving up the ghost, and seeking solace elsewhere. In fact, giving up the ghost seems to be more than a metaphor to describe me. I was becoming a ghost, physically at least. I was now indisputably skinny; my skeleton was visible through the skin which hung on my chest and arms. Losing one's eyebrows and eyelashes disrupts the look of the face far more than the loss of a few strands of thin, short hair should do. I looked like a ghost facially as well as in terms of body mass. On top of this, I was becoming pale.

Still I was not well enough to go to university, and I was missing one of the joys of my life, playing football. Soon, even walking became difficult. I would run out of breath within a few steps, my head would pound, and I would feel the sort of nausea which used to only come after a strongly contested fifteen hundred metre races. My limbs ached beyond my weakening and sagging muscles. They hurt to their very core.

This man started not only to look like a ghost, but to behave like one. Trust me, I wanted to do so much more, but found that the only solace from my discomfort would be to lie, prostrate, on the sofa for hours at a time. Only by wearing a baseball cap to cover my bald head and bare eyes could I make myself feel once more like a human being.

That is one of the horrors of cancer. It not only destroys your insides, but it reminds you, at every opportunity, that is doing so. OK, most of the symptoms I was describing were from the chemotherapy attacking the cancer cells, but also my own, healthy, cells were falling victim to its indiscriminate assaults. Like most people, prior to being subjected to it, I could understand that chemotherapy might not be a very nice thing to have to endure. But I had no idea at all of the reality of having that poison pumped into my body.

There were other symptoms as well. I often felt bloated, as though I had enjoyed an overly generous meal. Sometimes, I would fart uncontrollably. I was a set of mouldy bagpipes, all bones and baggy skin, emitting a mouldering sound which polluted the area around me. It sounds funny, now, looking back. It wasn't, at the time.

Without doubt, among the myriad consequences of taking chemotherapy, among the worst is the tiredness it induces. This is a tiredness so severe it hurts physically as well as emotionally. Often, it was not a tiredness which would be eased by sleep. I woke up tired, I stayed tired throughout the day, although most of that time was spent lying on the sofa, I went to bed tired, I stayed tired through the fitful, sleep disturbed night.

It is an aching tiredness, and all-encompassing one. Even the most everyday of tasks – attempting to eat, getting up to go to the toilet, getting dressed, could leave me completely exhausted. And remember, I was a young, fit twenty something. Six months before, I was working full time, studying long into the night, enjoying an active and fulfilling social life, playing football, going to the gym, playing tennis and other sports. Now, I was a wreck.

Cancer sufferers often point out to the loss of their hair as one of the most disturbing symptoms. It is the obviousness of it. It is a sign that hangs above your head saying, 'I Have Cancer'. It is a constant reminder that you are unwell, and not just with a cough or cold, but with a condition that not only threatens your life but changes it as well.

As a twenty-two-year-old, one of my most loved possessions was a leather biker's jacket. I didn't earn a lot of money as a legal clerk, but I was proud of that jacket. It was embroidered with a logo celebrating Guns'n'Roses. It was distinctive. But I couldn't wear it while my hair was falling out. In a way, that coat symbolised the healthy me, I did not want to tarnish it by putting it over the ghost I had become. Not that, of course, I could have managed to get outside for long to wear it. I tried to keep up appearances, I wore the baseball cap, tried to look normal. But everybody needs their image; even more so when they are a young man. Mine was gone, burst and hanging like a punctured bladder, eviscerated after just two months of chemotherapy.

With my hair, went my confidence. It seems silly, no doubt, to think of this young man facing a life ending illness but worrying more about his appearance. The shallowness of youth, and all that. But it was not the case. With my hair, went my manhood. My persona. I was changed. Although my pride made me keep it quiet, chemotherapy did not just eject the hair from my head and face, but my entire body. My legs, my chest, and beyond. All fell bald. It was as though some old, withered politician had admired Michelangelo's David, and employed a sculptor to carve a statue of himself. White, and naked. Hairless. Only, the sculptor he had hired was Ozymandias' artist, and he had seen the true passions of that politician. He bore witness to the old man's false pride. The statue he created was white, and naked, and bare and showed not the wisdom of age, but its weakness. 'Look on my works, ye Mighty. I despair.'

I was that statue, pale, thin, hairless. Old. In mind, if not years. I could hide the baldness of my body from others' eyes, and cover the lack of hair on my head and face with a baseball cap. I could not hide, though, the damage it was doing to my self-esteem, my confidence, my belief in myself.

The firm were understanding, Darren Loy was my immediate boss, he was a decent bloke. In the end, I needed to take 6 months off work. He, and the firm, stood by me throughout that time.

After six months, my chemotherapy stopped, and my hair began to grow back. But there was no relief in this. This is what cancer does to you. To any stranger, once the hair was back, I looked like a normal man in his early twenties. But I knew that this was not the case. That the hair on my head was different, that it was thinner, and felt different when I touched it. My post chemotherapy hair had a different texture, it was not mine. I had always been proud of my hairy legs. 'They are like your Uncle Fokrul's' my mother would say, when I wore shorts. Now, they were bare. The hair here did not return. My post chemotherapy self was a different person. To even the closest people to me, these changes were subtle. To me, they were distressing.

The trial had worked, I was free from cancer, but I continued to wear a baseball cap.

XXXXX

(I am aware that the description in this chapter is frightening. It is an honest account of the process of undergoing chemotherapy that I experienced. But my intention is not to frighten. My own chemotherapy was, at the time of writing, almost twenty years ago. Further, I was a part of a trial. Anti-nausea medication has come a long way; not everybody reacts as I did to the treatment.

I shall not lie; chemotherapy is not pleasant. However, it need not be as bad as the experience I underwent. The following chapter highlights some tips and ideas that have worked for some people. I wish I had known more about them in 2001).

Chemotherapy – The Advocate from Hell

Everybody's cancer is different. Every person reacts to the disease in their own way. Has their own lows, and – let us not forget – highs. But while the main purpose of this book is to tell my own story of dealing with the disease, trying to show that yes, cancer is frightening, but we can manage it, we can dominate it, it is also to try to give an insight into what we might face in the weeks, months and often years which follow diagnosis.

So, this chapter is a little more technical than those others we have encountered so far. In it, I will try to outline some of the generic physical issues facing patients undergoing chemotherapy, and then some of the emotional challenges of having cancer.

Chemotherapy Leaves You Prone to Infection

The chemicals we are pouring into our bodies are poisons. There is no getting away from that. Progress is already being made in directing those harmful medications at specific targets, and surely science will make us more accurate with our aim over time. But even the most advanced, laser fired rocket causes collateral damage, and currently chemotherapy is anything but laser directed. Medical practice dictates that these poisons will, in all hope and probability, provide more good than harm, and may be essential in a fight against the disease which is threatening to kill us. In no way whatsoever am I recommending here, or anywhere else in this book, that we do anything other than listen and consider our oncologist's advice.

But chemotherapy runs the risk of making us, in the short term at least, feel very poorly. I think that once we have that understanding, we can prepare ourselves mentally to stand up to what we are about to feel. However, as was the case in my situation, we might not quite be prepared for the extremes of nausea to which we find ourselves subject, but at least we are mentally on the right page. Equally, it might not be quite as bad as we fear; a bonus, if that is the effect that chemotherapy has on a cancer patient.

One of the effects of that poison is that our bodies become less effective at fighting infections. That means that we can fall very easily to infections that we might otherwise fight off. That is one of the reasons why cancer sufferers were listed on the Government's 'vulnerable' list during the Covid 19 outbreak. Physicians were left with the near impossible decision during the crisis of deciding whether a cancer sufferer was more likely to suffer worse from a pause in chemotherapy treatment or from catching the Covid disease whilst suffering from a weakened immune system.

However, cancer sufferers are more likely to find themselves open to a wide range of unpleasant infections when being treated with chemotherapy. Largely, this is because the medication reduces our numbers of white blood cells, which are our primary internal weapon we use to repel infection. But we can take control of our lives and take the front foot against the risk of infection. This involves nothing out of the ordinary, nothing that requires special knowledge of skills. Just common sense.

Among the measures we can take is the simple choice of **washing our hands regularly with soap and water**. One of the few silver linings of the Covid 19 outbreak is that washing our hands is something everybody now knows how to do. We can even cheer up the family (or neighbours, if we really go for it) with a loud rendition of Happy Birthday. Sung twice, of course, for maximum hand washing effect. We can further this basic hygiene tool by carrying **hand sanitiser** with us and using it when we are out and about. It is particularly important to wash our hands after going to the toilet, and touching animals – including pets – which can carry infections dangerous to us in our weakened condition.

We can show awareness of risk by **avoiding close contact with people who have an infection**. This includes even the common cold, as well as more serious conditions such as chicken pox, or the flu.

Every cancer sufferer (in the United Kingdom at least) is entitled to an annual *flu jab*. It is highly recommended to take up this offer. Flu has the potential to be dangerous in any case, but for a person undergoing a course of chemotherapy, it could be deadly.

A Cause of Anaemia

Anaemia is extremely debilitating. As we will see later, a key factor in managing our fight against cancer is our state of mind, our outlook and positivity. It is hard to be positive when we are afflicted by anaemia, because we live in a state of constant exhaustion. Anaemia is caused by a drop in the number of red blood cells, which carry oxygen around the body. Chemotherapy causes this drop in these cells. Once our number of red blood cells falls below a certain level, anaemia follows.

The symptoms to look out for include an *intense tiredness and lack of energy*. Chemotherapy in itself induces this uncomfortable lethargy, but with anaemia, the condition is exacerbated. A *shortness of breath* follows. This was something which I found particularly disturbing when I was taking chemo myself. The worrying feeling of *palpitations* can also be present. This is when we can feel our heartbeat inside our chest, and palpitations are often accompanied by a light headedness, and nausea is also felt. Palpitations are moderately unpleasant, but also worrying, because we are conscious that we are feeling them in our heart. Lastly, a **pale complexion** often accompanies anaemia.

The condition is usually mild, but it should never be dismissed as something we will just get over (although, in all likelihood, we will). In severe and unusual cases, the condition can become life threatening. A bad case of anaemia can result in insufficient oxygen being carried to our vital organs. Deprived of this, organs can begin to fail, and damage can be permanent. In the worst cases, our organs can shut down completely, and lead to death.

Therefore, whenever any of the symptoms described above appear, it is vital that we seek medical advice from our doctor.

Just as with infections, however, the good news is that we can take control ourselves and mitigate against the possibility that we will develop the condition as a result of the chemotherapy we are undertaking. Again, taking charge of our health is relatively easy. At least in theory, certainly, since the major way we can increase our red blood cell numbers is through diet, and when we are feeling unwell anyway, with nausea often present, the last thing we might want to do is to contemplate eating. Nevertheless, if we steer our diet towards one with a high iron content, we will help our body to increase the number of red blood cells it can create, since it uses the iron in our diet to form these oxygen carriers.

It is a common myth that to increase the amount of iron in our diets we need to eat a lot of red meat. Certainly, **beef, pork and lamb** are a ready and **good source of iron**, and for those of us able and willing to consume meat, we will get benefit from doing so. However, these days, for religious, health and social conscience reasons many people take the lifestyle choice not to eat meat. Fortunately, there are plenty of ways in which we can get iron into our bodies without resort to consuming animals.

Beans and nuts are an excellent source of iron. So too are dried fruits, especially **dried apricots**. Leafy, dark green vegetables are also an excellent supplier of this essential element. **Curly kale** is an acquired taste, but try it stir fried with a light sauce, and perhaps a few cashew nuts, and it becomes a bit more acceptable to most palates. But even if we find curly kale a step to far, then most people consider **watercress** to be inoffensive, and that too is an excellent source of iron. It also makes an attractive garnish! So, we can eat healthily but also attractively. Good news.

Lastly, **wholegrains** are good for finding iron naturally, and foods such as brown rice, or fortified breakfast cereals can top us up when our energy levels are sapping.

A Tendency Towards Bruising and Bleeding

Chemotherapy really does attack our blood supply. As well as launching an assault on both our red and white blood cells, it can also launch a broadside against the platelets in our blood. These colourless little cell fragments, sometimes called thrombocytes, perform the vital job of clotting when we are injured. Because chemotherapy can reduce the number of these blood cell fragments, we can find ourselves susceptible to bleeding from even minor injuries, and the bruising which results from blood seeping into surrounding tissue. So, even a small knock or bump might results in the kind of multicoloured temporary tattoo which tells us (and, if it is in a visible part of the body) our friends that we might not have conducted our movements as carefully as we could.

Of course, bleeding can become serious if a wound is deeper, and our platelet numbers have been devastated, because we may need medical help to staunch the flow of our wound in these situations. We should always inform our care team if we notice a lot of bruising, or if we start to suffer from severe nosebleeds, or bleeding gums, because these can be a sign that we have insufficient platelets in our blood, and we may need intervention to increase their number.

A Painful Mouth

A sore mouth is a common side effect of chemotherapy. It can seem a minor problem compared with the cancer we are fighting inside of us. But, really, it isn't. Because a sore mouth is debilitating, a constant discomfort and reminder of our illness. It is another factor which can wear us down. Typical symptoms of a chemotherapy induced sore mouth include a similar sensation to having burned it from eating food that is too hot. Mouth ulcers can proliferate, and because we are run down, they take a long time to heal increasing the danger of infection. We might experience pain when not only eating and drinking, but even when just talking.

Of course, it is important to eat well to maintain good health, and a combination of not being hungry because of the effects of chemotherapy, tied to a really sore mouth further making the thought of food unbearable can stop us from eating altogether. A dangerous outcome if not addressed quickly.

A sore mouth can affect how people perceive us. Whilst we might simply be quiet because to talk hurts, others might interpret this as us being depressed, in need of cheering up. When we just wish to be left to our own devices, because we are uncomfortable, well-meaning attention can become a pain.

A dry mouth is another symptom, as is an impact on our sense of taste. Bad breath too often accompanies this sort of oral discomfort.

But once more, we do not have to just live with such unpleasantness. By becoming proactive, seeking help and helping ourselves, we can reduce the impact of this side effect, and make life more tolerable.

We should make sure that we drink plenty of fluids, and often avoiding extremely flavoured foods can reduce our symptoms. Extremely salty snacks, spicy meals or sharp-tasting foods will exacerbate our conditions, while milder, more mundane flavours will be more easily managed.

The actual condition of a sore mouth does have a name – mucositis. Treatments for this condition are improving. Painkillers and medicated mouthwashes can help but it is always wise to seek expert medical advice with mouthwashes, since we do not want to use something which aggravates our discomfort. Therapies are developing which can stimulate healing through the use of low-level laser technology. Although this treatment is not widely available at the time of writing, it is growing in popularity, and it is worth pressing for if we are struggling with oral problems caused by our chemotherapy.

A Disappearing Appetite

One of the best ways of maintaining the energy to overcome – mentally and physically – the trials of chemotherapy is to eat well. Unfortunately, another side issue of the treatment is a loss of appetite. Once more, though, we can take measures to reduce the impact of this annoying side effect. Firstly, it is important to continue to consume plenty of fluids. This will help us to feel better; dehydration is a condition too easily achieved, and the associated symptoms – nausea, headache, lethargy, aches and pains, itchy dry skin – are all ones which help to lower our mood and negate our positivity. Both diarrhoea and constipation can be unwanted guests during treatment with chemotherapy, and neither contribute to the establishment of a healthy appetite.

But even though we might not want to consume large meals, we can adapt the way we take in fuel to make it more palatable. In doing so, we might even find that we eat more healthily, with all the attendant benefits that brings.

Firstly, it is important that we do not put pressure on ourselves to eat our 'three meals a day'. Well-meaning friends and relatives can easily add to our general sense of feeling unwell by, with the best intentions, urging us to eat when we do not want to. If we adopt the mantra of 'eat when we are hungry and stop when we are full' we will be well on the way to consuming enough calories. We must be careful of mealtimes becoming psychological problem spots where we feel we must eat a full meal because that is what is expected of us. Then, in addition to our new mantra, if we adopt the following guidelines, we will find that we are eating a perfectly acceptable amount and aiding our general well-being through doing so.

As a start, we ditch the traditional three meals a day expectation, and instead look to **eat more meals, but much smaller ones**. A large plate of meat, potatoes and vegetables can be really off-putting to a person who is not hungry. But, a small bowl of brown rice topped with colourful, vibrant, vegetables – stir fried and crisp; a fresh, light bread roll cut into a single open sandwich topped with our favourite filler; a few slices of an apple with some crumbly, piquant cheddar; a spring roll, freshly fried and crunchy filled. These little meals are more easily consumed, are tastier in their own right and, to be honest, much better for us than a carbohydrate heavy main meal.

Next, we seek to top up our daily intake with a range of **very light, very healthy, snacks**. A piece of fruit, a carrot stick, a couple of bread sticks dipped in some fresh, smooth, nutty humous, a handful of walnuts, a couple of dates.

On this point, it is also worth looking to balance our weekly intake, so we consume only **light meals on the days of our treatment**. These are the times when we are likely to be physically and psychologically most under pressure, and a lightly lined stomach here is better for us, in the long run, than having consumed a mighty breakfast or lunch. By eating lightly on the day of our treatments, we will hopefully feel less nauseous, and therefore able to recover more quickly and get back to a more normal diet for the remainder of the week before our next treatment.

Another factor which can reduce our appetite is the way we consume liquid. *Sipping slowly through a straw* enables the fluid to be absorbed more easily and reduces the feeling of bloatedness which often accompanies chemotherapy.

Changes to our Skin

We should be prepared as well for our skin and nails to change while we undertake chemotherapy. This does not affect everybody and can depend on the actual make-up of the chemotherapy we are undertaking. The most common side effect is for our skin to become *dry, red and sore*. This is naturally accompanied by an uncomfortable *itchiness*. Skin can become *sensitive to sunlight*, and may *discolour*, or become *patchy*.

Our nails, too, can be affected. They may become *brittle, or flaky*. Sometimes, *white lines* will develop running across them.

These conditions will go away once chemotherapy has stopped but can seem uncomfortable and unsightly during treatment. As always, worries should be shared with our care teams, who can offer creams which will offer some relief. We should try to cover up from the sun, and we can use moisturiser on our nails to help stop them drying out.

The issues described so far have been ones which are mostly physical in nature, although they inevitably impact on our psychological and mental health. However, there are other side effects which are much more to do with our emotional state and which, as such, are equally as distressing as the physical problems chemotherapy might bring.

Memory Issues

Although scientists are not fully clear why, sometimes people taking a course of chemotherapy may endure short term memory problems. Presumably, although not yet certainly, the stresses involved with dealing with the physical problems of the treatment, allied to the inevitable worries of coping with cancer, must play their part in causing this.

It is not unusual at all to find that our concentration and recall are both hampered during treatment. Undertaking simple, everyday procedures might also see an impact, with tasks taking longer than usual. Extra care needs to be taken when driving, and more time should be allowed to complete activities which normally we might do as a matter of course.

Again, we can alleviate this problem to some extent by making sure that we stay mentally healthy. ***Taking in a newspaper, getting our heads stuck into crosswords, sudoku, reading fiction and so forth*** – all of these can help to keep us mentally alert.

That Ravelled Sleeve of Care

Insomnia is yet another condition from which we might expect to suffer while undergoing treatment for cancer. Some people may find it difficult to get to sleep in the first place, others will wake up, and not be able to get back into unconsciousness. Shakespeare had it right when he had Macbeth fear for his sanity lest he should 'sleep no more'. (Mind you, he'd killed the King of Scotland, and so anything troubling his mind was entirely justified.)

Yet there really is little worse than staring at the walls in the early hours of the morning, unwilling to get up for fear of disturbing a partner, uncomfortable, tired and aching yet unable to find the comfort of sleep again. It is during those dreadful hours that worries grow and magnify, that we can feel at our lowest about our condition.

Insomnia seriously affects our mental health. In turn, that is very likely to affect our physical well-being.

If anybody could find a cure for insomnia, they would (rightly) become the richest person on the planet overnight. Stand aside Jeff Bezos, or Bill Gates, or whoever holds that accolade at the time of reading. The person who cures insomnia deserves every penny they earn. In the meantime, once more we can help ourselves to minimise the effects of this debilitating condition.

Routine is very important. Our body likes to know when it is time to undertake its normal activities, and so we should aim to get to bed at the same time each night, follow a getting ready for bed routine (whatever works for us) and also look to wake up at the same time each morning.

Relaxing before bedtime will help. However, one person's relaxation is another's cause of tension and stress. Some people like to read, others become wound up emotionally by the words they have just consumed. Some like gentle music in the background, others find a half-heard sound irritating. It is important that we relax with whatever works for us. Most people, though, find a warm bath will help them settle in for a good night.

Darkness and quiet aid sleep. Blackout curtains, an eye mask, earplugs or listening to 'white noise' will help most people. (There are plenty of apps – free ones – which will transport us to the smooth sound of an aircraft engine or the gentle patter of rainfall).

Again, it is a personal matter, but some people find that *writing a list of their worries* and concerns before going to bed helps them to lock them away overnight. Others, though, then spend time running the worries over in their heads, concerned that they have missed something.

There are a few 'avoids' which, again, will apply to most people but not everybody. Eating early, avoiding late alcohol, caffeine, nicotine, exercise and heavy meals in the hours before bedtime will generally help people to sleep better, and for longer. Similarly, it is best to avoid watching TV, using a phone or other technological device before attempting to sleep. However, this is a field about which there is much research taking place, and opinions are becoming better formulated.

If all else fails, it may be that our physician can recommend other treatments which will help us to sleep. Insomnia is a difficult problem to overcome, but not an impossible one.

The emotional issues that come with chemotherapy really cannot be underestimated. Forewarned is prepared and recognising in oneself that we could be heading on a downward trajectory towards depression may place us in a better position to tackle it. Fortunately, in a way unlike my experiences back in 2001, these days the stigma that comes with emotional difficulties is eroding. Slowly, for sure, but definitely. We increasingly recognise that suffering mentally is not something of which to be ashamed; to be scared, anxious, stressed is a normal human condition, at least in the western world in which we live, and talking about it is not only OK, but actually a positive step towards addressing the problem.

Macmillan Cancer support is a great place to start to find support groups in our local area where we can share our worries, getting support for ourselves and gaining the mental strength that comes from supporting others.

Talking is one of the best ways we can proceed when tackling our own emotional concerns.

However, for all the importance with which we need to treat the mental impacts of chemotherapy, it is the physical ones which might cause us the greatest immediate threat. Nevertheless, even then, although these physical consequences have the potential to be very unpleasant, mostly, they are not serious. The main exception to this rule, in cancer sufferers, is the onset of an infection. The seriousness of infection is magnified because our chemotherapy will reduce our body's ability to fight that infection. If we have the symptoms of an infection, we should always seek immediate medical advice. These symptoms include:

- A body temperature above 37.5 degrees Celsius.
- Or, one below 36 degrees.
- Breathing problems.
- Skin feeling hot to touch, or shivery feelings.
- Aches and pains, such as associated with the flu.
- A sore mouth, or pain when swallowing.
- Diarrhoea.

- Redness, swelling or discharge of fluid from a wound.
- Sickness

As can be seen, the impact of chemotherapy can be very unpleasant. It was especially so for me, and that was an important factor for what happened ten years later. But back in 2001, the treatment seemed to work. I had a career to achieve and a life to live. It was time to return to it.

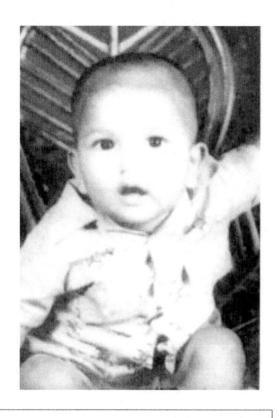

Always interested, even if it's just the camera. Me as a baby.

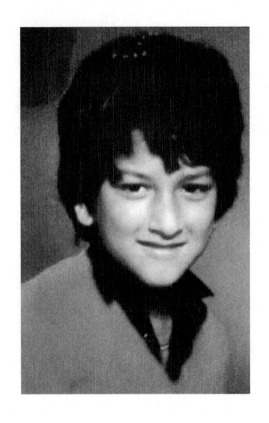

Aged about seven, photo taken at Regents Park School.

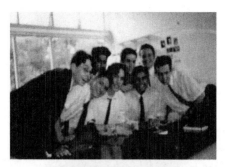

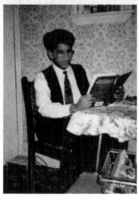

Studying King Lear at Camp Hill and with an encyclopaedia dad bought me when I was about 15.

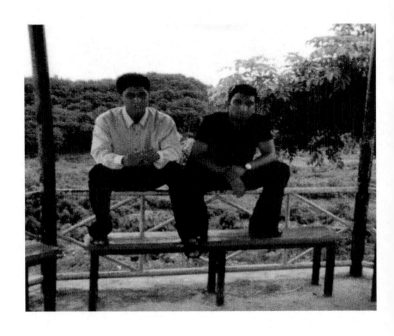

Above - in Bangladesh in 2001, with my cousin and canoeing pal, Sadat. I had just recovered from my first bout of cancer, and tragically, Sadat succumbed to cancer himself shortly afterwards, and died quickly.

Back packing around Europe, no prizes for guessing where this picture was taken.

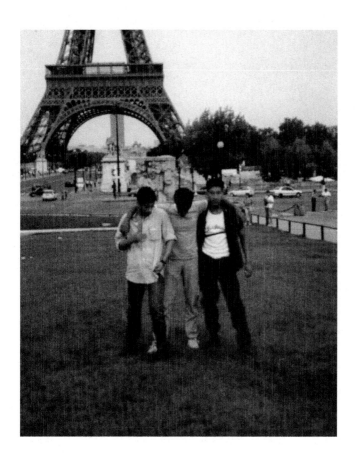

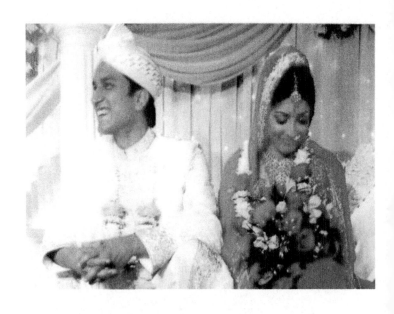

Our wedding in 2008. Beautiful national dress.

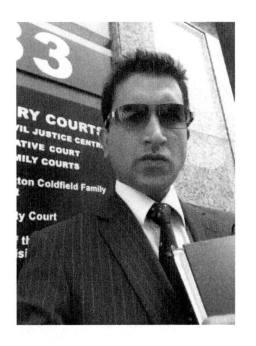

Outside court. Ready for another fight.

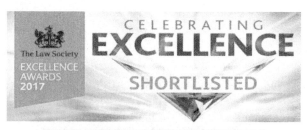

EXCELLENCE IN INTERNATIONAL LEGAL SERVICES

- Addison Aaron International Lawyers

There is always a great pleasure in being recognised by one's peers. Not bad, for a small, boutique firm.

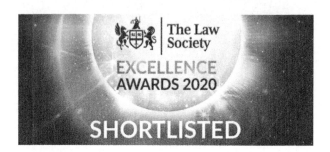

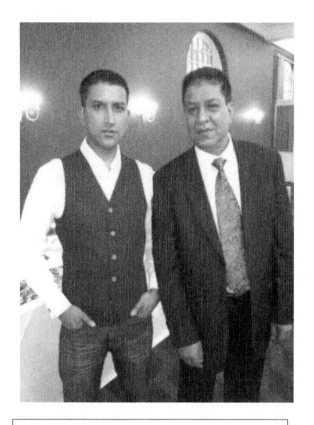

With dad. His work ethic is something to which I've always aspired.

Below, arriving at Cork airport for what would prove to be a frustrating case...

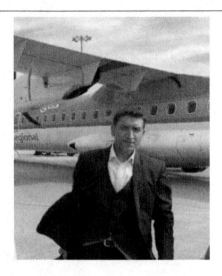

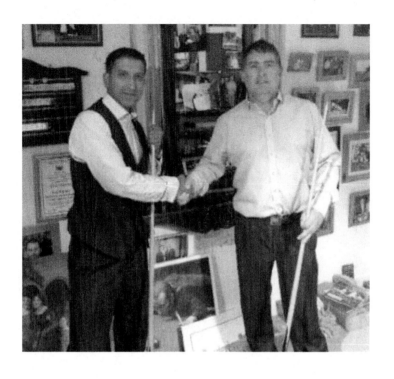

*... but at least I got to play some snooker
with Michael.*

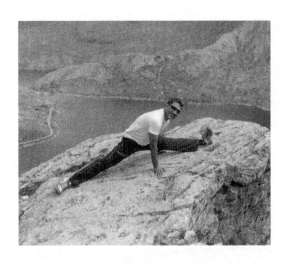

Keeping active...

Above – I've always been able to do the splits, but I haven't often had the chance to try them in such a beautiful setting.

Over the page top, on Snowdon once more.

Below, over the page, stretching out. There was no way I was going to allow cancer to define my life. I managed to combine my own checks on my health – if I could climb then I must be doing well.

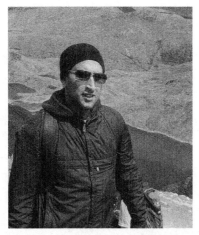

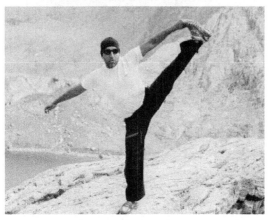

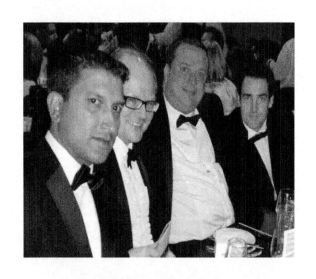

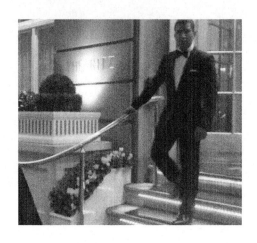

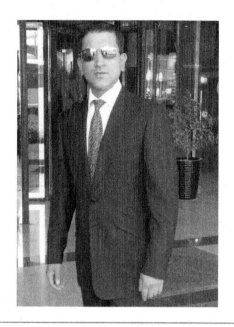

Above: On the way to meet a Sheikh.

Previous Page Top: Law Society Dinner 2015 – Me, David Jenkins, Mark Moss and Steve Brookes.

Bottom: Leaving the Ritz.

An International Lawyer

When my sister spotted the advertisement for an assistant at Dass Solicitors, I really fell on my feet. They were a leading commercial and tax law firm. They obviously saw something in me, because the firm sponsored me through my four-year part-time law degree at Birmingham City University. Working and studying simultaneously was a bit of a challenge, there is no getting away from that, but there is truth in the saying that the busiest people find the most time. I still managed to find the opportunity to spend nights socialising out and about around the country with friends. I still kept up my Sunday football, and played for the firm's team scoring all the goals with the outside of my foot.

However, before I do share some of my experiences of becoming and working at being an international lawyer, I think it is worth a short detour into some thoughts about the importance of education. I have already alluded to the fact that I was not the most committed boy at my school when it came to getting my head down and stuck into matters academic. I was a boy, after all, and other distractions took my interest. Getting laughs and having a good time being two of the most significant.

But education truly is a gift, a way to level up life's iniquities. Real education promotes understanding, not just knowledge. It is about sharing that understanding, employing it to improve the lives of others as well as ourselves. It is the nature of the society in which we live that to be respected, one normally needs to be educated. That is a controversial statement, but it is probably true. To lead a prosperous life, and probably a happy one, one needs to have studied and gained a good job. Education helps us to live independently, to gain freedom. It helps to protect us financially, and to live life on the front foot.

It is a subject about which I feel very strongly. I believe that it is only through education that social evils such as poverty and racism can be eradicated, although that is long journey to undertake. A necessary one, though. Parents have their part to play, to provide and expose their children to the appropriate education for their age and stage of development.

Life is about competition. That cannot be avoided. There are winners and losers. It is important to inculcate children into this inevitable fact from an early age. It is also through education that the rights of women can be promoted. There remain societies where women continue to live as second-class citizens. Education helps to address this. As Nelson Mandela said, 'Education is the most powerful weapon which you can use to change the world.'

Education was what allowed me to survive cancer. Not just the education of my oncologists, but my own. 'The roots of education are bitter,' said Aristotle, 'but the fruit is sweet.' That was certainly my experience when it came to tackling my own disease. But this chapter is about my career as an international lawyer. It was education (with a little help from my sister) that led me on my career path, but also education that helped me to find that law was the correct path for me.

I strongly believe that when young people, those at the age of eighteen or so, finish their formal schooling it is quite likely that they will still be uncertain what job they should pursue. There are many ways of achieving results, which is a big lesson to learn in business. Similarly, there are many ways to discover which career is right for us. Studying at university for three years can really help to formulate a person's thinking. We might spend forty-five or fifty years working at a career – more the way retirement age keeps being pushed back. It is only right that enough time is given to deciding what that career might be.

A good understanding of accountancy is a must for a successful businessman or entrepreneur. Similarly, sales and marketing must be priorities. We could have the best business ideas in the world, selling the finest products at the most attractive prices. Hopeless, though, if we cannot get our message out, or recognise how to turn those products and services into profit.

But if university is one way of gaining that grounding, a good method for helping young people to decide what they wish to do with their lives, it is not the only route a person can choose. My philosophy is a simple one, really; we can do anything we think we can do. If we want to improve our lives, we can.

Education. There is nothing more important. Which leads me neatly on to the genesis of my career in International Law.

There is a lot to be learned from starting at the bottom. And that was something I certainly did. 'Office Junior and Tea Boy'; if I had an office back then, that is the label that would have sat on the door, most probably in the basement at Dass Solicitors. Much of my early time was spent in reprographics. Which is an over grandiose way of stating that I spent hours at the photocopier, running through bundles of papers. I spent two years doing this, and the only way to mitigate against the boredom of such work was to read some of the documents I was copying. Retrospectively, this provided excellent preparation for the role I fulfil now as an international lawyer. By reading these documents I gained an insight into many different aspects of the legal profession. I suppose that the technical term is that I was broadening my knowledge through a wide range of current, active case studies. It is hard to think of a better way of learning. Brains are at their most potent in the late teens, and I absorbed such a range of material that I simply learned and learned.

As my time at the photocopier progressed, I found that I was becoming particularly interested in accounts, and soon I find myself with a more specific role – Accounts Assistant. A far more impressive title for the imaginary sign on my imaginary office door. My experience was broadening out. Next, I was promoted into the criminal law team, where I became a legal clerk. During my time here, I worked on two murder cases, particularly unpleasant ones since they involved a baby and a small child. That kind of work was fascinating, on one hand, but at the same time extremely disturbing.

I also became involved in a high-profile case which involved international, cross border enquiries and carried global implications for airline safety. The case, the Stansted Hijacking incident, involved the landing of an aircraft by terrorists. The plane had originated from Afghanistan. It was a complicated case, the hijackers holding the plane on the runway of Stansted airport for more than three days. The men involved were eventually convicted of hijacking and false imprisonment and sentenced to five years each in jail. Their sentences were later overturned when it emerged that the trial judge had made an error in summing up.

The case rumbled on, with it being determined that the hijackers could not be returned to Afghanistan because of the risk on their own human rights of doing so. Later, it was ruled that they could stay in the UK on the basis of a 'discretionary leave to remain', which guaranteed them freedoms such as being able to work in the country and choose their own place to live.

Although it was not a route into law I had explicitly planned, studying for my degree whilst working on the job was, in retrospect, an excellent move. It gave me real life experience, not just academic study. The cases in which I was involved where genuine, contemporary issues, and not just old studies which had already been analysed to death. Of course, there is value in the study of law as an academic discipline; indeed, such an undertaking is essential to any person seeking to make a career in the profession. But to do so whilst gaining daily, first-hand, experience might have been extra hard work at the time, but it was essential in launching my career. Unlike those who study purely at University, I was able – on a daily basis – to test the theories which I was learning about on live cases.

I spent time in the company commercial department during my early years. It was then that I had the chance to study under the expert eye of David Jenkins. Here I was involved in both the setting up of companies, and also dissolving them. I began to understand the process of completing statutory books. I even worked, for a time, on a bankruptcy case that had spanned an incredible twenty-four years.

I graduated in 2002 with a law degree and four years of experience behind me. Anybody who assumes that lawyers immediately step into the world of high earners should take a rain check. My pay was extremely poor, and having struggled by for four years, as well as spending close to nine months side-lined by cancer, I decided that I needed to try something else.

I took a job for a sales company which involved travelling from door to door selling gas and electricity. I was probably the best qualified door to door salesman in the nation. Incredibly, I found this work to be far more lucrative than the legal profession, and I was soon earning three times the sum that I would draw from my previous employers. The money was incredible. To a young man I felt as though I had made it. A manager at the business would be on a salary of £65000 per annum. It was an enormous amount back then, and a sum magnified by the eyes of a young man. It started to become my goal to seek that management role. I was sure I could do it and applied myself intently, for a while.

After five months I started to see through the job. I really did have other ambitions than an involvement in sales. Soon, the idea of becoming a manager and entering the daily grind of an unchanging rat race lost its appeal. The money might be good, but there was more to life than this. I decided to leave, and joined a recruitment company, working on placing candidates in jobs in the engineering and construction industries.

It might seem like I moved around unable to settle down, unsure of what I wanted to do. But, in my defence, I have a couple of arguments. Firstly, I had focussed totally on my legal career for four years. Yes, I enjoyed an active social life during these times, but like so many other young people I needed to try new things. To gain new experiences. Secondly, I had recently undergone a life-threatening disease, the treatment for which had made me so ill, feel so bad, become so afraid of the regular chemotherapy treatment sessions that I was unsettled in my mind. I was entering a stage through which most people pass – sometimes earlier, sometimes later – and to which my specific circumstances made me particularly vulnerable.

Not that I regret any of the decisions that I made. Regret is a very negative emotion. It should have no place in our brains or our hearts. That recruitment business gave me my first experience of leadership...and I loved it, I met Khalid the warrior. I found myself advising companies on matters such as growth and succession planning, and this work planted the seeds of my wish to set up my own business. These dreams grew quickly, and within six months I had left the recruitment world and had achieved my dream of setting up on my own. With enormous excitement I began selling telethon products. The business really took off, and very quickly the money was pouring in. I lived like a prince. But I was heading for a fall. I was placing an enormous amount of trust in my sales manager; I was still young, and naïve in many ways. This manager, it turned out, was inflating both his salary and his sales figures, making excessive claims about his success rates.

Of course, everything imploded. His breach of trust left me scarred, but more worldly. I had learned a lesson, a painful one admittedly, but one that would serve me well. No regrets.

By now it was 2005, and having tried my hand in recruitment, sales, business management and leadership I felt that I was gaining a good context upon which to base my future career. I decided that a return to study was called for, and once more worked full time in a law firm while studying for my legal practice qualification that would allow me to practice as a solicitor. I began to gain international experience since 2006, I have worked in more than twenty-five countries, with a mixed caseload of dispute resolution work (more on this later).

Then, in 2009, my friendship with David Jenkins — I had worked under him at Dass Solicitors while studying for my initial law degree — bore further fruit. We decided to set up shop together, and founded Addison Aaron, a commercial and international law firm.

Addison Aaron (Addison, means the son of Adam, and Aaron was the brother of Moses and his advocate, Aaron also means a mountain of strength). I bet you didn't know that?

When we started, we set up on Church Street in the centre of the city, next to the old eye hospital.

Birmingham is England's second city. It lies close to the centre of England. It is home to a major international airport, it is circumnavigated by three motorways – the M6 to the north, the M42 to the south and east and the M5 to the west. It exists smack in the middle of the industrial heartland of the country. Its extensive canal network makes it the Venice of England. That it has grown to be a major city is remarkable, really, since it is not close to the coast and nor does it have a major river flowing through it. Yet, from the 14th century it has grown to be a city of significance. These days, it is home to well over a million people – two and a half million if we extend its boundaries to the built-up area of the West Midlands. That is more than three times the size of the next biggest city – Leeds, and six times bigger than Manchester.

Yet would any stranger to the country recognise this. The aforementioned Leeds and Manchester, along with Edinburgh, Glasgow, Cardiff, Liverpool and perhaps even the likes of Bristol and Sheffield enjoy higher profiles. Therefore, it makes me proud that I can represent Birmingham on the international stage: 'raising the city's flag as a centre of excellence in international dispute management, commercial, fraud, insolvency, corporate and property law.' That was written in the brochure of The Birmingham Law Society Legal Awards 2015, when I was a finalist in the category of International Lawyer of the Year. (The accolades have continued, which makes me very proud. As I write this, in the Covid infused days of summer 2020, I have just been notified that Addison Aaron have been shortlisted by The Law Society of England and Wales Legal Awards 2020 for "Excellence In International Legal Services." Such recognition does not pay the bills, but it helps to keep the company in the public eye. And, I have to be honest, it is a fine feeling to be recognised by one's peers, in whatever walk of life we choose to follow. These awards are the Oscars of the legal world and they mean so much to me, I would like to thank everybody that has supported me in this journey.

In 2015, I was involved in a contested probate dispute worth £1.7 million which was cutting across three jurisdictions – England, Switzerland and India. It was a ground-breaking case, one of the first in the High Court to test the newly implemented Inheritance and Trustee's Powers Act of 2014.

At Addison Aaron, as I have said above, we are delighted that we have won numerous Birmingham Law Society Awards. Among the hundreds of legal service providers across the west midlands, we were finalists in 2015, 2016 and 2018, whilst in 2017 we made it to the last stages of the competition for The Law Society of England and Wales Legal Awards for "Excellence in International Legal Services." This was a huge achievement as this category is open to firms all around the country and some overseas law firms. I have already mentioned our success in 2020, hopefully we will go on to win this year.

I am proud to say that that I have worked across well over twenty five jurisdictions. We advise multi-billion-dollar companies in the Middle East, to assisting individuals on as far as Australia. As well as being heavily involved in high profile cases which cut across international borders.

Not that it always works out as we hope. I remember once getting an urgent call. A potential client in Ireland had a problem but could not find a solicitor to represent him locally who could help him win his case. A friend of mine, Michael, heard about the client's problems, and recommended he got in touch with me. He did, and I was happy to help.

I flew out to Cork, met the client and within a relatively short period of the time I had a solution. I was growing a reputation for the lawyer to turn to when nobody else could help. Unfortunately, this client did not continue with his case much further.

Still, I got to spend some time with Michael, which was great. He's a big snooker buff. Waistcoats of the famous from the game, line his loft, which accommodates a full size table. Whether it's snooker or law, being a rocket always helps. We played a few times, I lost. Losing sometimes helps the formation of the spirit. At least, that's what I told myself. When it came to snooker, Michael was in another league.

Which I suppose leads on to another point to make for would be lawyers. Not that we need to hone our snooker skills, but that it is not always as financially rewarding as might appear from the way we are presented on TV and in film. I love my job; I adore building a team – no lawyer can handle a case on their own, a team of experts needs to be created to support them – I adore winning cases or finding settlements for my clients.

And the money is OK. I wouldn't deny that. But it is not amazing. We do not all drive around in a Bentley, although I have owned a Porsche I say with a smile. I deal with a lot of big money cases. Even so, because a battle might be over millions of pounds, that does not mean that my fees are anything like that. And what lawyers are able to charge is spread thinly. The essential team has to be paid. A lawyer's insurance costs are high; the risk of being sued ourselves is an ever present cloud.

There are partners, secretaries and consultants to pay and various other costs.

We occupy offices in a splendid grade two listed building in the centre of Birmingham. Being an international law firm means, we work around the clock, from England to the four corners of the world. Sometimes I have to take calls very early in the morning or late at night, as someone has just woken up in Japan.

So my message is to go into law because you love the idea; the British judicial system is one of the best in the world, perhaps the best. Join it because you want to be a part of it, to do good and not for the money. If you do become a solicitor because of thoughts of becoming rich, then sadly you are entering the wrong profession, for the wrong reasons.

Work hard at school and university, and you can be part of a profession that is a joy to belong to. The money is OK, it will be a bonus, not a driver of your career.

But enough lecturing. For a boy from a town in Bangladesh, my career as an international lawyer really has been invigorating. I advised a shipping and trading company in Dubai, which was the victim of a $2.9 million cyber fraud. This case involved tracing, freezing and recovering monies worldwide. Cyber-crime is on the increase and businesses need to take extra precautions.

I have worked on a number of other cases in Dubai, including advising a $4 billion turnover company, who were seeking to recover monies from a company based in the UK. I remember going to London to serve a statutory demand, and then up to Great Yarmouth for further investigations.

The firm has advised on divorce and financial disputes in England, France, India and Australia. It really amazes me, how the name of a small firm like ours, gets around.

A banking dispute I did was a particularly complex and potentially a sad matter. The client was an elderly lady, a mother who had guaranteed business debts of her children but had done so without receiving proper advice. Her home was facing repossession. I had to take on the case at short notice, and spent days working through the paperwork with a fine-tooth comb, the office becoming my virtual home for a while.

When I had met her children, a couple of men in their fifties, I remember the expression on their faces. These were men who were distraught about how things had worked out. They had not intended, of course, to land their mother in this impossible position.

In fact, the first time I met them, they took one look at me and asked me my age. I was thirty two at the time, but looked ten years younger. 'He's just a baby,' I could see the thoughts rushing through their minds.

They decided I was not for them, went elsewhere, and lost the case. It was only then that they came back to me. Now the matter was much harder, since a decision had already been reached. One I would have to overturn. Still, banks are heartless institutions. The old lady was ill, and did not really understand what was going on, and they were about to make her homeless did not bother them in the least. There is plenty of evidence that forcing old people out of their homes can lead to drastic physical and emotional consequences. They did not care.

I was not going to allow that to happen.

I managed to identify the flaws in the bank's case, and delivered these eloquently in court. My preparation in the office, being key to saving this lady's home.

Winning a property investment dispute case in Cyprus against a national bank, was very important for my client. We had to work really hard, going the extra mile, successfully removing charges on his property in London. I nearly got to go to sunny Larnaca. Being an international lawyer means that sometimes you have to travel overseas, it has its ups and downs, I guess you get some me time but you can become lonely, it can get tiring and really boring waiting around airports.

I worked on one occasion for a company in the Ukraine. This case was an international insolvency litigation, resulting in enquiries in the USA and Singapore. In a matter that crossed into France, I acted for a group of property investors from Liverpool.

I had another case not dissimilar to the one involving the old lady and the threat to her home. A client was recommended he speak to me when he was about to lose his home. He had contacted numerous solicitors and barristers, and none were interested in a case it seemed certain they would lose.

Then his insolvency advisor said he'd heard of a firm in Birmingham who took on the impossible. Addison Aaron. I built my team, and together we persuaded the judge not to act too presumptively. I was new to the client, I explained. Give me time to investigate properly. The Judge did, and I managed to find a lawyer in London to join the team.

Together, we discovered that there was more to this than met the eye. No wonder his creditors were desperate for a quick resolution. At Addison Aaron we rarely go to court, as we tend to settle matters at the earliest possibility.

I have had other cases of this kind. My time working for Dass had been based around VAT work, but I had been occasionally side lined into general crime, especially fraud, and from there into civil litigation.

That is how I built a reputation for tackling civil, commercial and criminal matters.

Perhaps the most unlikely victory I ever secured for a client involved a complex case of bankruptcy involving 'John Doe'. This client was made bankrupt and the bank had an interim charging order on his house. Normally, the rule is that such a charging order will fail on bankruptcy because it has not been made permanent. However, the Insolvency Act provides that if a person has gone deliberately bankrupt, or borrowed money fraudulently, then those circumstances allow an interim charge to be made permanent. The problem is that a bankrupt person is not allowed to defend his own rights, he has no locus standi. Therefore, the bank believed that their application to make the interim charge permanent could not be opposed by John.

My network of lawyers advised that the case was one we could not win, but they had overlooked something important. We investigated and discovered that the bank's evidence was fraudulent. My client won the case. Several lawyers had refused to help, too worried about their own reputations to assist a client in their search for justice. Once more, the point that everybody has the right to defend themselves, and to receive professional support in doing so, has to be stressed. It is one of the foundations of our justice system. Some people in the British system need to remember that fact.

A man in Coventry was about to lose his home. The bank were happy to take it. But when I spoke with him, it turned out that the bank had no right to the home, because the man did not even own it. It was his father's home, and that of his disabled mother.

I do not take people's homes, I save them.

So, as you can see, setting up and working for Addison Aaron has really opened my horizons. David and I founded the company, David is now a consultant, and Steve Brookes my new partner. Together with our dynamic team, we deliver exceptional results in the most difficult cases across the globe. Proof that serious cancer scares do not have to become life dominating even if, as we shall see in the next chapter, they inevitably become life changing.

Indeed, a touch of brashness never goes amiss. I was involved in an employment matter where two sisters had been unfairly dismissed. The company was being represented by one of the largest law firms in the world, an everyday name which has a reputation for being the best of the best.

Christmas was closing, and I didn't want this matter rushed through the tribunal before the holiday period, when people's minds would be on other matters, and the case could become a bit of a lottery.

I phoned this international monolith of a law firm, and spoke to my opponent, whose toffee nosed responses seemed to indicate that he did not expect to be contacted by somebody such as me, a guy from a boutique law firm in Birmingham.

'We've got a tribunal coming up,' I told him. 'And you're going to lose this case, because I am the best.' (I had found his attitude so disdainful that I was becoming quite angry.

Perhaps he did not fancy having to share a court room with me, because the next moment he was ready to negotiate a settlement for my clients, which they were delighted to receive.

As a final note for my work as an international lawyer, I have been fortunate enough to become involved in some cases defending celebrities from drink driving issues. This is a whole new world, one where the lurking presence of the press adds extra pressure. I am proud to say that these cases were successful as well, resulting in the termination of the prosecution. I can offer a little more information, without identifying the accused, in this matter.

When the media star approached me, he had been already been turned down by a number of advocates who felt the case was hopeless. Yet the accused insisted on his innocence. I told him that I could investigate matters fully and give him the opportunity to state his position. The clerk of the court, on this occasion, was sadly typical of some people who work in the system, who appear to make an assumption of guilt before the matter has even been heard. We needed to seek a lengthy stay before the case came before the court because the star had committed to a long tour and if this were to be cancelled tens of thousands of members of the public would have missed out on seeing their hero. The fact was, if my client were to be found guilty, a custodial sentence was not out of the question.

'I know what you're doing!' shouted the clerk at me when I announced that we would be pursuing a long date for the hearing. Was there an element of racism there? Was it just that this clerk was sure my client was guilty, and we were simply putting off the inevitable? Have we reached the point where clerks to a court decide on the guilt or innocence of the accused? I don't know, but this court official was hardly upholding the need for neutrality essential to any system of justice.

Anyway, the clerk was required to take himself off the case, because I applied the pressure. This was a tactical manoeuvre on our part, because it was going to be a very difficult case to win. Normally, there would be only one hearing, but we managed to put sufficient doubt in the justices' minds that we forced through four separate hearings, until we terminated the prosecutions case.

Sometimes, I suppose because it sells papers, there is a feeling in these cases that the big names get away with their misdemeanours because they can afford to hire top lawyers and can pull strings. As if they are not Mr, Mrs or Miss Joe (or, I suppose, Jo) public. That may happen on occasions, I would not know. However, just because a person is a celebrity does not automatically impose an assumption of guilt. A drink driving celebrity is entitled to just the same level of legal support as me or you, and they are also just as likely to be facing a false charge to which they have every right to fight and, if they are not guilty, to have their name unblemished by the accusations levelled at them.

In some ways it would be great to share, in terms of general interest, more details of these cases, but of course, to do so, would throw away the accused persons' complete entitlement to anonymity, and their right to put a difficult time behind them. Keeping matters confidential is another key role for any lawyer, international or otherwise.

I wanted to include this chapter for many reasons. High in the list is the fact that cancer does define a person. Not completely. We can still live very successful lives during and after the course of the disease. Yet, however much we might want it not to do so, it does change us, and (as we shall shortly see) becoming a cancer survivor marks us out. That identifying feature is meant to be admirable, but just as a facial scar might tell of a heroic act, mostly those of us who have survived, and continue to survive, cancer, just want to get on with our lives. To be normal. To live like anybody else.

My career as an international lawyer, and it is with no false modesty that I can say a successful one as well, gives proof to the concept that it is possible to move on from cancer. To embrace a career, a family, an existence. Cancer is terrible. But it is a step-in life, one which if our temperament is positive, does not have to become anything more than a very temporary barrier to our ambitions.

Mind Games

I can only speak from experience and personal research. But the psychological threat of cancer challenges the primacy of its physical one as a cause of suffering in patients. Receiving a diagnosis of cancer has been likened to hearing news of a bereavement. I can understand that. It is as though you have been physically assaulted, the wind is knocked out of you. Your mind moves into a state of blurred confusion.

Those early moments are ones in which it can be extremely difficult to identify the feelings that are passing through your brain at such intensity that they jumble together. If we were a plug socket, it would be as though a surge of power has suddenly passed through us – unexpectedly, however well we prepare for that session with our doctor or nurse – and blown our system. We do not function. For a moment, we are hopeless. Useless.

That state passes quickly enough. Our bodies are good at coping with shock. But another problem soon raises its head. We may begin to identify the feelings we have; but they can be myriad. Anger, guilt, blame, distress, a need to crack jokes, a need to cry, confusion, fury, sadness, failure…we are all different. But even though we can soon separate our emotions into clear, if connected, strands a new issue emerges. Can we honour those feelings? Can we pay them the respect they deserve? Because, if nothing else, they are honest emotions. Ones which deserve our time, deserve to be heard, to be explored and then, utilised in our best interests.

Clearly, obviously, a diagnosis of cancer is frightening. Fear and worry are inevitable and appropriate responses. Working through them, embracing them, can turn them into positives. Recognising and respecting our emotions can lead to us reducing stress. It can, if we are honest with ourselves, lead to improved mental health; that, in turn, can help our physical well-being.

Yet it is human nature to judge ourselves. For most of us, we are our biggest critics. We are harder on ourselves than anybody else would ever dream of being. We set ourselves huge expectations, and we come down on ourselves even if we achieve them. Success is failure unless it is a bristling, bursting, beaming success, exceeding all expectations. By contrast, take successful professional athletes, people whose own mental strength must be supreme if they are to make it to the top. As the audience, we watch an Olympic final and are disappointed if our contender does not win a medal. Actually, we are often disappointed if they do not win gold. But consider the interview with the athlete afterwards. Frequently, they are beaming with pleasure at their fifth place. Fifth place in an Olympic final. Of the almost eight billion people on the planet, only four are better at that event! An incredible achievement, if we think about it. *They* have thought about it, and they recognise their astonishing success as such. But for most people, with their unrealistic expectations of themselves, and what constitutes success, they regard that fifth place as nothing.

Certainly, winning the battle with cancer is like winning an Olympic gold, but too often our expectation of ourselves is not just to cross that line first, but to do so without enduring pain, doubt, fear, worry, mood swings, depression and deep troughs in our state of mind along the way. All of these are emotional states from which we should expect to suffer, from time to time. If we are ready mentally for the battle ahead, if our expectations are realistic, but ambitious, we are halfway to winning the fight.

There will be times when our life seems completely without point or hope. If we know those feelings are going to arise sometime, we can prepare for ourselves, fight them, envelop them and defeat them.

There are, however, some conditions which we have to meet in order to be prepared for the emotional battle ahead.

We Must:

- **Be kind to ourselves;** we are suffering from a serious, let us be honest, life threatening illness. The treatment we choose to undertake could well be unpleasant (although this is a subject we will return to later). It is important therefore that we do everything we can to make life as pleasant and as comfortable as it can be. We should take up offers from friends and family to help us out – they would not be made if they were not well meant. Where possible we should give ourselves treats. The temptation can be to put ourselves through some kind of personal austerity experience, as though telling ourselves that cancer might think it has made our life bad, but we can make it worse still. No, we should be kind to the most important person of the moment. Ourselves.

- **Not judge ourselves for our emotions**: As we have said, there will be bad times. There will be times when we are unjustifiably angry, miserable and even unpleasant to be around. It will happen. People understand. We do not make that worse by coming down on ourselves because we cannot remain upbeat through every moment of every day. There is a beautiful couplet in James McCauley's magnificent poem 'Because'. It is not about cancer, but these lines have special resonance for the importance of avoiding judgement of ourselves.

'Judgment is simply trying to reject
A part of what we are because it hurts.'

•   **Understand that our hope and confidence will increase:** It is a natural condition to feel a sense of loss when we first receive a cancer diagnosis. The thought of living under the heavy skies of cancer, and the prospect of treatment can overwhelm even the strongest person. We can feel like giving up hope. However, these emotions can, and do, pass. There are measures we can take to help speed up that process:

○   **Live in the present:** the distant point at which we will become cancer free can seem so far away, and that is daunting. Try to live in the now. Set extremely short-term goals. Make those goals realistic and achievable. Look only to the present and the immediate future. Make a list of two or three targets to achieve each day. Physically tick them off at the end of the day. Such successes will make us feel better. Do not let regrets of the past haunt us, do not allow our thoughts to wander into the long-term future.

o   **Surround ourselves with positive people:** There is a theory called the law of attraction. Simply, it states that we surround ourselves with people who reflect our outlook, and that outlook is then magnified by the presence of such people. Thus, if we are determined to be positive, we will attract people who are positive, and that will help to improve our mental and emotional health, because we will become ever more affirmative about our prospects.

o   **Ensure we have a strong support network:** Friends, family, neighbours. They will *want* to help. Let them. But do not forget the importance of the expert network there to support us as well. Our healthcare team. Engage with them, and they will respond. If they do not, insist on a change.

o   **Consider counselling:** Counselling is a high-quality skill. Top counsellors hold advanced qualifications, and really do have expertise in helping us to face our challenges and develop resilience and mental strength. There are many support organisations, local and national, which can provide guidance, or put us in touch with counsellors appropriate to our needs. It is not a weakness to seek mental health support, it is a strength.

Cancer's Victims are Manifold

Suffering from the disease is terrible, there is no getting away from that. It is best to be honest. Few, if any, people will take a diagnosis in their stride and remain unaffected by their condition. Once we accept this, we have made the first step towards coping with the condition. However, it is not just cancer patients who become cancer victims. Family and friends are also deeply affected when a loved one is diagnosed with the disease.

Family will worry about losing us. How they will cope with our suffering. Their lives will change as ours evolve, and that can be unsettling. Peoples' reactions will vary on discovering that their close friend, or brother, son, mother, father, sister – whoever – has contracted the disease, and faces months of treatment. Especially given that there is always a possibility that the final outcome may not be what is wanted. Cancer can be, and sadly, sometimes is, a fatal disease.

This uncertainty means that there is no one way that people will deal with the news of their loved one's situation. People who love us, and whom we love, might become incredibly angry at us for contracting the disease. They may become overprotective, they may refuse to talk about our condition, or overtly recognise that we have cancer. *Every person deals with their reaction to the news in their own way.*

That can be hard for us to take. We may feel that we not only have to cope with the ravages the disease, and possibly its treatment, but also deal with our friends' and family's reactions to the news. We have to face the probability that somebody along the way will say something that offends us or hurts us. That is not their intention. Merely, it is just their own inability to understand their own emotions about the news that has upset them deeply.

It can be very hard to cope with the fears of others when we are trying to cope with intrusive fears of our own. That is true whether it is we who have the disease, or we are trying to support somebody else who has contracted the condition.

It is fine not to know quite what to say when we discover a friend, or family member, has cancer. If there were an easy response, we would all use it. I suppose that the best reactions come from those who listen when a friendly ear is required, and who stay positive throughout. When we have cancer, much of the time we want to be distracted from its pervasive influence, we want to do things that are fun, have laughs, be positive.

Most of us will have, at some time, worried about contracting cancer. We will have spied a lump on our bodies, a mole that is benign, an illness that won't go away and wondered. We try to think what we will feel like, how we will react, were we to be given the news we so desperately do not want to hear. Naturally, the reality of actually experiencing the disease, or seeing it take hold of a close friend or member of our family, is likely to be very different from our perception of what might happen. Nevertheless, those trial feelings are important. Because, *having considered the horror of the disease places us in a better position to be a great friend and support when a close one to us succumbs.* More than this, we are all survivors in one way or another. Not everybody, thank goodness, contracts cancer. However, bereavement, loss, failure, the end of relationships – each in their own way helps us to build up resilience and puts us in a stronger position to support others when the disease strikes them.

We must be aware of passing on, or receiving, the myths of cancer. The truth is we should work with our medical teams, the experts in the field. Of course, it is useful to become experts on the condition ourselves. Understanding helps. Later on, I will explain more of my own experiences of the disease, my own approach to dealing with it. Whilst that might seem, to some, unorthodox, I state now, and I will reiterate later, at all times I operated with the support of my medical team. Everybody knows somebody who has, or has experienced, cancer. Their experiences will not necessarily be the same as our own.

Cancer is Personal

There are two very distinct elements to all cancers. There is the disease itself, which takes many different forms, and passes through numerous stages. Then there is the person whom the disease is attacking. We are all different. It is unreasonable to expect that we will all respond in the same way to the disease. Cancer really is personal. What has worked, or failed, for another holds only partial significance for our own reaction to it.

Within those elements exist numerous more variables; two people in stage 2B of a particular cancer variety could show markedly different symptoms. On a molecular level, every cancer is unique. Oncologists vary in their approaches. This is not to say one method of working is better than another, although finding an oncologist whose approach matches your own needs is a very good ambition to hold.

We may get the disease, but the last thing we are likely to want is to become defined by it. Cancer sufferers are people with an existence beyond cancer;

we want to enjoy our life beyond the disease and have the limits the conditions places on it as minimised as is possible. People with cancer frequently live full and fulfilling lives. Sadly, of course, sometimes those lives are shortened thanks to the disease eating away at their insides. But we should never forget that we can always win the battles against cancer. Frequently, and ever more often thanks to medical advances, that means we win the war as well. Some people do not, tragically. But most still want to enjoy the life they are living to the fullest extent possible.

Cancer helps people to gain perspective. To see what is really important and what is less so. Important to them, of course, and every single person's priorities are different. That is why cancer is like real people – individual and unique. There is no average cancer sufferer, no typical patient.

Consider a person who has caught the disease early. Whose prospect of survival are extremely high and who can be treated with the minimum of invasive surgery. For that person, their cancer remains the worst they have ever had. The same fears are present as they would be, if they have been diagnosed with advanced lung cancer. In both circumstances, worry, stress and terror will each be present at times. And there will also be occasions when happiness floods through the victim. As a friend of the sufferer it is important to recognise this. Knowing that, for example, our mother's condition is curable, and is very likely to be dealt with may be a comfort to us. There will be times when it is on no comfort whatsoever to the person suffering from the disease. Times when an arm around mum's shoulder is the best support we can offer.

Therefore, it follows, that there is no particular way to *feel* about cancer. However we respond, that is fine. Our responses are up to us and others must respect that. Most probably, they will. More to the point is that we must respect our reaction ourselves. Achieving that is sometimes the hardest challenge.

The Changing Mental Impact of Cancer

'You're looking well, how are you feeling?' That is the sort of loaded question cancer sufferers often face. But those who pose such questions, well-meant and showing an interest, should pause a little before asking it the next time. Anybody who is ill will feel pressure to answer in a positive way, in so doing making the questioner feel better, and also avoiding the inevitable (but usually reasonable) instruction to 'stay positive'. However, there is more to a response than that. Because, how people feel with cancer not only changes week to week, or day to day, but as quickly as hour to hour or even minute to minute. Physically and psychologically.

We are concerned about the latter of these at the moment, and any pause before answering the question might be interpreted as negative. Even if the response is *pause – 'Not so bad, thanks'* the answer could be taken to mean the opposite. The power of the pause is considerable; but can also be mis-read.

Because such a hesitation could well be genuine. 'Well, I felt really positive when I woke up, but over a cup of tea the thought of next week's chemo started to hit, and I was quite miserable. Then I had a walk, and felt better, but at the moment, I'm quite worried...' Not the sort of answer the questioner probably wants to hear.

'Yes, but how do you feel at the moment?'

'Good. No, I can feel the stress coming on.'

It is completely normal to expect our mood to change quickly and illogically when we have the disease. Reason and logic are thrown out of the window where this condition is concerned. It is far from unusual to get the results of a scan which throw up real concerns, yet to feel positive, even joyful. Equally, a day which should prove a challenge – perhaps a chemo day, for example – might sometimes feel like a walk in the park. Then, twenty-four hours later, finding the effort to get out of bed might be beyond us.

So, it is extremely important to try to feel positive when suffering from cancer. But at the same time, the inevitably negative, unpleasant feelings which will flit from time to time must be embraced just as readily. It is perfectly fine to feel down. Perfectly reasonable to cry. Perfectly acceptable to shout and scream, if that is where our mood takes us. Honouring our feelings, allowing a sense of grief in when it is knocking at the door serves to enable us to feel even happier when it finally decides to leave, and we close the gate behind it. Whether its stay has been for a week, a day or just a single minute. Enjoy it when it is gone, respect it when it is present.

The Loneliest Disease

Another important aspect of cancer which not everybody always appreciates is the loneliness of the disease. Even for those with the strongest support network, there will be moments of considerable isolation. For all the help we receive, cancer is a solo journey, a dangerous, challenging trip we never sought to embark upon in the first place, and which now we must complete, wherever we joined the path.

Where family and friends understand that sense of isolation, they are best placed to give effective support.

Many who suffer from cancer see friends disappear. There is a saying that real friends are the ones who stick by us when we are in trouble. That is true, but only to a certain extent. Even dear, dear friends can find the challenge of supporting their closest companions an insurmountable challenge. These people do not become less frequent visitors because they are fair weather friends. No, the difficulties of dealing with a changed mate can just be too much. That might seem weak. How can the challenge of coping with a friend's cancer compare to coping with our own? A fair enough question, but that is the nature of cancer. It impacts on more than those it invades, and it does so without logic or predictability.

Nevertheless, when friends, or family members, seem distant or become so, that can have an enormous psychological impact on the victim of cancer. Our impossibly lonely journey has become even more isolated. In such circumstances, the words of a friend take on even more importance. Simply being told that our spouse, or parent or child loves us, and will always love us means so much, does so much good, even though saying might be hard, especially when that loved one is very ill.

Being aware of the loneliness of cancer is important for those who become part of a support network. Never take for granted that your support is understood, and therefore needs not be spoken.

Yet although a support network of family and friends can help to alleviate loneliness it cannot take it away. It is wrong to try. The words that often cause most harm are the best meant ones. 'I know how you

feel,' or 'I understand what you are going through...'
How can a friend understand what we are going
through when we do not understand it ourselves?

Becoming a part of the support network for a
cancer sufferer requires a thick skin. We can be the
closest person to the unfortunate with the disease,
their spouse, their parent, their closest, longest friend.
Yet it is not unusual that people with cancer choose to
share their innermost fears with strangers. Support
groups do not contain our closest friends, but that is
sometimes what makes it easier to speak honestly to
others in the group.

The lonely journey of the cancer patient is an
oxymoronic one. Yes, there are times when the
loneliness comes from direct isolation. For myself,
during my first battle with the disease, those times
were especially during the nights when I could not sleep
but was fearful of disturbing others. So many dark
hours spent just thinking; and middle of the night
reflections always suffer from the intrusion of
blackness. A second aspect of the loneliness is that very
alarming sense of not knowing how we actually feel. If
we cannot define it ourselves, how can others have the
slightest idea of what it is like, suffering with the
condition?

But finally, there is the very business of being a
cancer patient. We have our normal lives to lead; we
probably enjoy more visitors than when we are well.

Then, on top of that consider the additional duties and chores which the cancer patient faces:

Hospital appointments – not just with our oncologist but with other members of the team who are treating us, including the many times our specialist wants us to get a second opinion on a medical decision; not only do we have to attend these appointments, we have to get to them, make them and accommodate them in our lives. We will be regular visitors to our local pharmacy, and there is the strong likelihood that we have regular chemotherapy appointments to fit in and recover from. Then there is the research we want to carry out, surfing the internet, reading pamphlets from our doctor, sharing stories other sufferers, online or in person. These are just the administrative extras that enter our lives. We must tackle these while suffering the physical and emotional rollercoaster that cancer brings.

Understanding this can help friends and family to appreciate the loneliness those with cancer endure. Education is enlightenment.

The Pain of Cancer

We have focussed, rightly, in this chapter on the emotional challenges of cancer, both to those who suffer from the condition, and also those who are close to such patients. But we should not lose sight that cancer can hurt, physically. Pain amelioration is a science that is improving with leaps and bounds. There is no need to suffer the sort of agonies under which patients struggled in years gone by. Nevertheless, cancer might sometimes hurt, and pain makes anybody miserable. Particularly when it is long lasting, and no end is on the horizon. That sort of pain can make us tetchy, unreasonable. Our closest friends and family understand this, and do not take it personally.

Certainly, some drugs might cancel the pain but offer other, unpleasant side effects. Research suggests it is the fear of pain which is one of the most corrosive aspects of having cancer. People worry about addiction and can put pressure on themselves to be 'brave' through pain. Evidence shows that most late stage cancer sufferers are under treated when it comes to pain relief. That is another, personal, challenge we have to overcome on our long and endless journey.

The problem, though, is that any journey through cancer is a long one. And also, with regards to the majority of cancers, one without end. Even when our current condition is cured, the risk is that the tumours may return. That chance can be very small, and regular check-ups can help us to ensure that we can catch a relapse early, but few people can claim that they *did* have cancer. Rather a person *has* had cancer, the present perfect continuous form of the verb indicating that the chance is there that they may return to becoming a patient in the future.

Imagine that. Knowing that we are never going to be completely cured of the threat to our lives. We become cancer survivors, defined by the disease from which we have suffered. Imagine how much a cancer patient wants to get off of that never-ending journey, if even for a day.

The phases patients will go through can be distressing. There is the inevitable anxiety about regular check-ups. The fear that grows as the time for the hospital approaches, and the wait for the hopefully good news that we remain clear of the disease. But, sometimes, for some, the words we hear will not be good. We have a diagnosis. The cancer has returned.

The process begins again. Treatment. Worry. Isolation. Hopefully, recovery. Until the next appointment. Sometimes, of course, the news never becomes good. For too many, still the cancer progresses. Treatment becomes about slowing the canker's spread. Searching for treatments to extend life. Deciding the point at which treatment must stop, and the inevitable accepted. Preparing for the end of life.

Yet even in these darkest of times, the peculiarity of the disease – or perhaps it is the human state – remains. Some days will still be filled with joy, some moments funny, sometimes good. The human spirit is astonishing. It keeps going to the end.

Cancer Changes Us

That is a fact and cannot be avoided. We are changed in the eyes of others, and therefore – inevitably – in our own perception. We don't stop being our child's father, our subordinates' boss, the guy or girl who enjoys a pint. But we add to our list of personal titles 'cancer survivor.' Often, in many people's eyes, that is an 'achievement' which is pushed further up our personal list than we choose ourselves.

But there are other changes. Fears which have been pushed to the furthest corners of our adult lives – ones we embraced as children, like fear of the dark or being seen as different - come back to haunt us. They leave blemishes on the inside as obvious as the changes to our hair, or the scars from operations to remove tumours.

Two things I have noticed from my own cancer are that every time I shave, I see the scar of the biopsy I had back twenty years ago. It is a daily reminder of what I have been through. It does not go away. I am also not as strong as I used to be. I was always a bit of a show off; right back from those days learning martial arts, I have been able to do the splits, and I still can. But I am not as physically strong as I once was.

We change spiritually as well. Cancer brings death closer to us, in perception if not always in reality.

But although cancer changes us, often the way we evolve is for the better. It makes us review our mortality, our place in the universe. It can impact on our personal faith.

It changes our perspective on life's everyday stresses. We become far more tolerant and understanding of the pressures on our friends and family. We become more attuned to their moods and worries. At the same time, it is not unusual for cancer survivors to be less tolerant of others annoyed by the minimal irritations of life; the inability to find a parking spot just where we want, the need to miss a favourite TV programme or football match because of a prior engagement or demand from work.

Things that seemed important before our diagnosis no longer are. Our priorities change. Our relationships change. Our role in our family and friendship group changes. Everything, in fact, changes to some extent or other.

That is the damage that cancer can do. But it is also, conversely, an unexpected benefit it can bring. Nobody chooses to live with cancer. The positive changes that can follow its invasion are ones we would rather reach by another means. But we should never forget, millions suffer from the disease, cope with it, grow from it and defeat it, at least to the extent of keeping it at bay. My own journey is one such account. Rarely do we hear of any but the ones closest to us of those multitudes of stories. That does not mean that they are not taking place. Daily. Continuously. Victoriously.

The Lymphoma Litigation

The human mind is a strange object. It can absorb overwhelming evidence pointing towards an undeniable conclusion, but if it does not like that conclusion (or, conversely, likes it too much) it will do everything in its power to convince that another explanation exists for whatever the matter in hand might be.

In September 2011 I was in London on a case at The Royal Courts of Justice. It is one of the largest courts in Europe. The courts within the building are generally open to the public with some access restrictions depending upon the nature of the case being heard. It was that day I felt unwell, with some discomfort in my lower back as the client and I went for a meal at a restaurant after the court hearing. Looking back I am sure that was the start, the return of the cancer.

It was in October 2011 that the mosquito bite appeared on the side of my neck again. Mosquitos are not especially prevalent in London or Birmingham, and particularly rare when Autumn is turning towards winter. Unlike most mosquito bites, this one grew of its own accord, swelling until it could not be ignored. Tooth infection. I made an appointment for the dentist, told him about the niggling pain in the bottom left hand side of my jaw and allowed him to carry out a full examination, including x-rays. There was nothing wrong with my teeth. In my heart, I knew that this was the case.

Even though it seemed unquestionable that the cancer was returning, I still remained in a sort of fear induced semi denial. I remember going to see Uncle Shahed at his house.

He knew straight away, as he must have recalled seeing that lump back in 2001 or probably because I was so conscious of the lump on my neck that I ducked my head down inside my collar, so I looked like Elvis. 'Don't tell me that shit is back again,' he said.

My mind was filled with the agonies of chemotherapy I had endured last time round. I was older now, in my thirties. I was a partner in a legal business that was growing more successful by the day. But the lump continued to grow. My cancer had returned. There really could be no doubt.

The logical part of my mind got to work. It seemed like I faced three options. I could die from the cancer; I could submit once more to chemotherapy, but I was increasingly sure that this time that would kill me if the cancer didn't, or I could become proactive myself in my treatment. I began to read. I absorbed everything. I would go to my dad's house at nine o clock at night and research on the internet until three in the morning. In that first week I think I probably read for eighty or more hours. The power of education.

I guess that I was researching as a way to avoid dying, and perhaps more relevantly, as a way to avoid chemotherapy. My spirituality is an important part of my life. Muhammed the Prophet (PBUH) advocates the benefits of black seed oil. It was a start. Another natural benefit which many articles said brought benefit was carrot juice. My wife went out and bought a juicer for me, one of the best £40s she ever spent I would say.

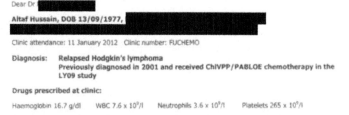

Dear Dr ▮▮▮▮▮▮▮

Altaf Hussain, DOB 13/09/1977, ▮▮▮▮▮▮▮▮▮▮▮

Clinic attendance: 11 January 2012 Clinic number: FUCHEMO

Diagnosis: **Relapsed Hodgkin's lymphoma**
Previously diagnosed in 2001 and received ChIVPP/PABLOE chemotherapy in the LY09 study

Drugs prescribed at clinic:

Haemoglobin 16.7 g/dl   WBC 7.6 x 10^9/l   Neutrophils 3.6 x 10^9/l   Platelets 265 x 10^9/l

The recent left upper cervical biopsy has shown that Mr Hussain has relapsed Hodgkin's lymphoma. He was very upset to hear that he has relapsed disease this morning. He is due to have a staging CT scan on 19 January.

As it is over 10 years since his original diagnosis, I think that if we confirm that he has stage IA disease, that treatment could be three courses of ABVD chemotherapy, followed by local radiotherapy.

He had his sperm banked before his original treatment back in 2001, and in fact has been to The Women's Hospital recently regarding fertility investigations, and apparently his current sperm count is very low.

I have arranged to see him again in two weeks' time, when we should have the results of the CT scan, and can make a more definitive plan for his treatment.

Kind regards
Yours sincerely

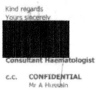

Consultant Haematologist

c.c.   **CONFIDENTIAL**
Mr A Hussain

This letter of January 2012 confirms the worst news.

Depending on how many of the life-giving root vegetables I had, I would take the drink in a cup or glass and enhance it with a teaspoon full of black seed oil. It is recommended to take this supplement in two doses, half a teaspoon in the morning, and half a teaspoon at night. I was taking three spoons a day, in three cups of carrot juice. I had no proof of whether it would help. But I was doing something. I was taking responsibility. I was using my education.

I continued reading, I continued taking this self-composed treatment. I went for my biopsy. This was in December of 2011. To my naked eye and persuasive mind, it seemed as though, by this stage, the tumour on my neck had stopped growing. It was hope. A glimmer. Nothing concrete; nothing definite. Perhaps the intrusive lump was nothing to worry about. In January of 2012 I was back in hospital, and the news was not good. The biopsy had revealed that the Hodgkin's lymphoma was back. In my heart, my brain – in fact in every part of me – that was the news I was expecting. It was still a shock. I was devastated although it was the doom-laden proclamation I was certain I would be hearing.

It was the start of a really terrifying time. My wife and my sister Forhana were my moral support, accompanying me to the hospital.

Diagnoses:	**Nodular sclerosing Hodgkin's disease stage 2b treated in 2001.**
	Recent relapse with localised stage 1a disease in left cervical region.
Previous treatment:	**ChIVPP PABLOE in the LY09 trial**
MDT decision:	**To proceed with 3 courses of ABVD chemotherapy followed by radiotherapy.**

Results: **Haemoglobin 16.9g/L**   **WBC   5.5 x 10^9/L**

              Platelets 212 x 10^9/L   **Neutrophil 2 x 10^9/L**

It was a pleasure to see Mr Hussain in today's outpatient clinic. Thank you for your recent letter about the treatment for his condition. I had another discussion with Mr Hussain and his wife. His sister was also present during our consultation and one of our SpRs Dr ████████ I have explained to him that the research shows that 3 courses of ABVD followed by radiotherapy will give him a high chance of being cured and if he does not have any treatment and the disease progresses then obviously the chances are much less. As a compromise at the end Mr Hussain said that he will see our oncology consultant Dr ████ for consideration of radiotherapy as he is very, very reluctant to have chemotherapy.

This letter from early in 2012 shows the worry I had about embarking on another course of chemotherapy. My doctors were understanding and sympathetic.

I was petrified of a second course of chemotherapy. Perhaps, in some ways, the time lapse between now and the first time magnified the horror of that previous experience in my mind. All I could think about were the injections, the embarrassing, painful bloating and attendant wind. The alternate constipation followed by diarrhoea which I remembered cutting me in two, such was its ferocity. Overarching every stinging anxiety, like a nebulous devil spreading its cloak, shadowing all, I feared the vomiting. The terrible, never ending, nausea. It is a strange, and

149

probably fairly British trait, that the human animal finds bodily functions amusing, especially when they go wrong. Everybody has suffered from stomach troubles in their life; this aspect of cancer treatment is like that, only continuous and ten times worse. OK, you have to laugh. I didn't feel much like that then.

'We should start the chemotherapy again as soon as possible,' said my oncologist.

'Let's see how it develops,' I replied. My oncologist agreed to grant a temporary stay from the chemo. Another appointment was made, and again I took my wife and sister with me to the hospital. (They accompanied throughout this difficult time, for which I am eternally grateful. The fact that one of the doctors was a Greek God, an Adonis, was, I am sure, a complete irrelevance in their decision making).

The choice at the hospital was the same as before. Chemotherapy. To start as soon as possible. I declined the option. My family were sure that I was wrong and should take the chemotherapy path.

'We cannot just wait and watch,' urged my doctor, my sister, my wife. I had almost settled on the fact that they were right, and I would have to subject myself to chemotherapy.

The letter below did not copy too well, but shows the problems we were facing.

I was very pleased to see Mr Hussain in the clinic today, along with his wife. It is very difficult to convince him about the best option for curative treatment for his disease. I can fully understand this, given that he is completely asymptomatic; he has no residual palpable disease at the scar site and he had such a traumatic time with his chemotherapy the last time, most particularly finding the hair loss and nausea a real trial.

He is fully aware that our recommendation for treatment would be three cycles of ABVD chemotherapy followed by radiotherapy. He has now seen Dr ██████ team, although I have not got a clinical letter from them, but I think one of their thoughts was that if we did a PET scan, we could at least get as much information as we possibly can to assure ourselves that this is truly localised disease and they could then give localised radiotherapy on the understanding that this is sub-optimal treatment.

I did offer the support of a psychologist today, just to try to work through some of the previous difficulties with treatment and try to get around some of the fear of pressing on with best treatment. Mr Hussain is adamant that he does not want to be referred to a psychologist.

I tried to explain to Mr Hussain today that as he is adamant that he will not have chemotherapy, if we do, do a PET scan and this shows that there is more disseminated disease that we would be left in an extremely difficult position, as the only option for treatment would be to consider a chemotherapy based treatment plan.

The doctor went on to say:

Given the difficulties we are facing here I am happy to ask our radiology doctors to authorise a PET scan and we will take things from there. I have arranged an appoint (sic) for him in three weeks (sic) time, when I hope very much we may have been able to organise this and get some form of result to inform our decision making.

'The other possibility is radiotherapy,' said my understanding doctor, when I hesitated once more. I was as petrified by that alternative as the chemotherapy. Possibly more so. I had read about the possible side effects of radiation. It was not a route I

151

would permit. It would have to be the chemotherapy option. Life was operating in a sort of blur, but through those mists occasional shafts of light would shine; they did not bring good news. Each time my mind cleared, the thought came in that there was a fair chance I was going to die. I was a young man, in the prime of life. I had just set up my law firm, Addison Aaron. I loved my parents, my sisters, my friends. Most of all, I had been married only two years. My wife was a black country girl, brought up in the West Midlands borough of Smethwick and an accountant by trade. But back then the last thing I wanted was for my wife to watch me as I died, prostrate on the sofa, unable to move, unable to function.

At the same time, the thought that she would have to share the appalling journey where I lost my hair, my eyebrows, my confidence was equally as bad. But the calls from the hospital kept coming in. I needed to start treatment. I think that this was the darkest time of my life. Worse than the first bout of cancer, and all the suffering and discomfort of that. Because I had even more to lose now. But still I researched, seeking out any lead which could point to the science which, surely, must somewhere point to something that could save my life.

'You have to go to hospital for your treatment.' The comment was bouncing in my head, propelled by friends, colleagues…family. I reacted with anger, with hurt. I gave every excuse I could think of to avoid the inevitable, to put it off, to buy myself a bit of false time. Still I consumed my black seed oil and carrot juice. Fervently, almost addictively. And I researched.

In fact, reading was what I did. Dozens of articles, pages of information. I began to see that diet could be a major contributor to tackling this disease. From the never-ending tunnel which headed down into a pit of pain, misery and, very possibly, death I began to see a light. A third route, outside of chemotherapy or radiotherapy, barely visible - but there. A risky one, never fully explored in the scientific world. But different people had entered that alternative tunnel, exploring in the darkness at least for a distance. Trying new ideas, new ways. Some, it seemed, bore fruit. Diet. This could be the escape for which I was looking. I might have to climb that path myself, like a mountaineer finding a new route to the mountain's summit. But alone, without the support of companions, or equipment. Just myself, my belief and my hope.

Because although I was surrounded by people who loved me, who would do anything they could to help, I had cancer. I had the disease that makes you alone. But knowledge gives strength, and slowly, very slowly, my confidence began to return. The darkest hour had past and although it was still night – the dankest, longest night – I knew that dawn would come. Eventually. The worry started to fade.

Worry is a cancer in itself. It invades every moment, even when we are sleeping. At night it is what leads to bad dreams, to restlessness. During the day it is the all-pervasive stalker. Even when, for a glorious moment, it fades into the shadows, it comes back suddenly, hitting hard to make up for the moments it was away. Worry invades, it takes hold, it spreads. Slowly, imperceptibly, until it has consumed our entire bodies. It is a sustained fear, and it feeds from indecision. 'Shall I do this? Is it worth the risk? What if it goes wrong?' Worry stems from equivocation, an unwillingness to make decisions. This leads to an unsettled mind, and an unsettled mind is helpless.

Most people suffer from this to some extent. Most of us lack the will power to reach decisions promptly, and then to stick by them once they are reached. I did not reach a quick decision. But, finally, I swallowed hard and made my choice. I would reject radiotherapy. I would reject chemotherapy. I would deal with my cancer through diet. And positive thinking. My friend Dr Hak arrived at my house. I showed him in, told him about my research, explained what I intended to do.

'That's absurd,' he said.

Abdul Qayyum an audiologist, my long standing friend, called me one day. He had spoken with top oncologists in London and told me to speak with them. They too explained the science, what worked and what

154

did not. Statistically, they explained, my best chance of survival lay with chemotherapy. I do not question their judgement; they are experts in their field. They know far more than I. Except, my cancer was attacking me, not them. I knew that chemotherapy was not right for me – not at that time. I am not saying it would not have worked, sent my cancer away for a second time. To make such an assertion would be pure speculation.

But I had done my reading. I had chosen my path. I would stick to it.

I have a sweet tooth. I adore chocolate, I love cookies. Caramel cake can send me into raptures. But my next dietary change was to stop consuming white sugar. This meant missing out on these treats. Yet in my mind tackling this disease which was attacking my body once again came down to a binary choice. I would kill it before it could kill me. I had read in some journals that cancer feeds on sugar. If I stopped consuming this far from nutritional substance, I would starve the cancer. (OK, sugar tastes really good, but there's more to life than that. Literally.)

Mind you, my self-imposed abstinence from the sweet stuff was mitigated to some extent by my love of honey. That too would become an integral part of my diet. However, I came across this beautiful elixir not directly as a result of my cancer. It was 2014 and the symptoms of Hodgkins Lymphoma were in abeyance.

Then, I began to develop a pain in my abdomen. It was just below my ribcage, slightly to the side of centre. For a while, this ever present discomfort scared me to death. I really believed the cancer had returned, and not only returned, but spread to my stomach. My confidence evaporated, and I forced myself to my GP expecting to be sent straight to the hospital for a confirming X ray.

Fortunately not. H-pylori was the culprit, a fairly common bacterial infection which causes stomach pain and other unpleasant symptoms. The relief that the problem was relatively benign was considerable, but having committed myself to treating cancer through diet, I was disinclined to start pill popping now.

My doctor suggested he would send me to the hospital for them to put a camera up my backside, when I heard that I ran a mile. I went back to my research, and discovered that honey was an effective anti-bacterial agent

I started to take it, neat, two or three tablespoonfuls a day. Within 2-3 months, the H-pylori was gone, and my symptoms were relieved.

It turned out that my sister also suffered from H-pylori. I told Salina to take some spoonfuls, but she does not listen to me. Younger sisters, what can you do?

And, of course, I had the advantage of the lovely sweet taste of the nectar. That might have been that, but during my research I had come across the role of honey in Islam.

There is a story. A man goes to the Prophet (PBUH) and complains of stomach pains. The Prophet (PBUH) advises him to take honey. He does, but it does not cure his pain. He returns to the Prophet (PBUH) and says that the honey does not work. This is repeated on more occasions, until in the end the man is told that he must take honey, and believe in that honey. He does, and the pain goes away.

So, I discovered, honey was already an important element in my religion. Almighty Allah makes reference to honey in the Holy Quran in Surah al-Nahl (The Bee). '...there issues from within their (bees) bodies a drink of varying colours, wherein is healing for people: verily in this is a sign for those of thought' (16:69). Honey is a healing for mankind, I discovered.

The Prophet Muhammed (PBUH) said: 'By Him in whose hand is my soul, eat honey, for there is no house in which honey is kept for which the angels will not ask for mercy. If a person eats honey, a thousand remedies enter his stomach, and a million diseases will come out. If a man dies and honey is found within him, fire will not touch his body.' He also said of the sweet nectar, 'The condiment of drink is honey. It guards the heart and drives away cold from the chest.' And, on another

157

occasion, 'He who desires protection, let him eat honey.' And 'It sharpens the sight and strengthens the heart.'

The Prophet (PBUH) was himself fond of the life enhancing substance. A'ishah said that the Prophet (PBUH) would drink a glass of water sweetened with honey every morning. He told his followers, 'Do not refuse honey when it is offered.' He was fond of a drink made of milk, honey and raisins.

There is good, scientific evidence backing up the use of honey as a medicinal purgative and healer. Its medicinal value is promoted by many scientists. It is a traditional medicine from many cultures, dating as far back as the ancient Egyptians. Laboratory tests demonstrate it is effective at hampering the growth of the likes of E Coli and salmonella, although whether it does so in humans is not scientifically proven. It is also a demonstrated source of antioxidants.

However, honey should not be given to infants certainly up to the age of one. This is because of a risk of botulism unless the honey is cooked to kill the bacteria which might potentially exist within it. For older children and adults, it is believed to offer the following health benefits:

- It eliminates the mucus which can build up in the lungs; as such it is a particularly useful additive for those with colds and fevers. Just consider how many over the counter cold medications include honey in their constituent parts. That is not just for the soothing sensation the viscous liquid offers.

- It aids health in the digestive system. It removes parasites and helps to prevent bleeding. When I was basing my cancer treatment on control of my diet, it was vital that my digestive system was not compromised, honey helped to achieve this.
- It helps to boost the immune system. We are learning more and more about how everyday foods can help us to stay fit and healthy. Honey is the great grandfather of this movement.
- It softens our faeces, helping to avoid constipation.
- Honey has very effective anti-fungal, anti-bacterial and anti-viral capabilities. This is always of importance if we are to stay healthy but is especially so if we are suffering from cancer, when we are more susceptible to disease and infection than is normally the case.
- It detoxifies our bodies. This cleansing not only make us feel better but improves our digestion and helps to prevent infections.
- It is a balm to the liver and kidneys, helping to keep both functioning effectively.
- It makes our skin shine, look healthy and younger. We could fall into the trap as seeing

this as merely providing a boost to our vanity. But when suffering from a major illness, this benefit really comes into its own. We have seen that the psychological impact of cancer is one of its most negative facets. Yet if we look good, both to ourselves and to others, that can help us to feel positive.

(These benefits of honey, and many others, are confirmed in a number of sources.

The Prophet (PBUH) also recognised that honey can be beneficial when both consumed or just simply applied to the skin. It helps our bodies to control our temperature, it contributes towards keeping our bowel movements regular. When Queen Elizabeth I used it to clean her teeth, she knew more than mocking modern historians might sometimes recognise. Not only did it help her teeth to shine and to freshen her breath, but it brought all the myriad benefits mentioned above. It is also believed by many to help regulate menstruation, as well as performing the function of keeping the hair silky and strong.

Take a look through the higher end pharmacies and health shops that proliferate in the more up-market shopping arcades, and we will see that honey-based products are prominently displayed and are big sellers. It is a major presence on our supermarket shelves, although we have to be careful with cheaper products that the goodness has not been refined out. In many ways, honey has become the unspoken gem. However, that could become dangerous, because its measured sweetness, flavoured with the plants the bees from whom it came visited, could lose popularity, replaced in the diet of the young by nutritionally devoid, obesity inducing product that is refined sugar.

Our taste buds become acclimatised to whatever they are exposed. Refined sugar is cheap. We know from the obesity crisis gripping the western world, and the pressure on the Government to tackle sugar consumption in the UK, that this problem is already widespread, especially among the less affluent sections of society. Whilst honey is not a luxury food in terms of price (although it is in terms of nutritional and health-giving benefit) it is a lot more expensive than refined sugar. We become used to, perhaps even dependent upon, the harsh, sickly taste that refined sugar in a product instils.

If honey ceases to be a regular item in our shopping baskets, we are throwing away one of nature's most beneficial products. One that nourishes, is medicinal, a flavoursome drink, a sweetener and a cream to top other foods. One that helps to regulate, protect and cure our bodies.

It became a major part of my diet as I tackled my cancer.

I reviewed Mr Hussain in the haematology outpatient clinic today. He remains well with no history of E symptoms. He tells me that he is recently back from a holiday in Spain.

On examination there is a node palpable in the neck, he showed me the area where he had his lymph node biopsy. His abdomen is soft and non tender with no organomegaly.

He remains well and can continue to work. I have planned to review him back in our clinic in six month time.

The sort of news I wanted to hear when I set out on controlling my diet.

Still, despite my benediction to the glories of honey, it took an enormous amount of will power for me to give up refined sugar. I remember Uncle Shahed offering me a chocolate, the temptation was so great. But like a recovering alcoholic offered the smallest tumbler of sherry on a visit to his maiden aunt, one morsel could be enough. All my effort would be wasted if I climbed back aboard the sugar train. If I was going to defeat this aggressor inside my body, I needed to stand firm. In fact, I quit sugar for more than two years. I was on a mission; one that it was in my own hands to deliver. By January 2012 I was treating myself with my diet of no sugar and with huge quantities (relatively) of carrot juice and black seed oil. My tumours seemed to have stagnated. They were not going away, but crucially they were not getting any bigger. I am not going to say that my fears had receded; I was still extremely worried, but I also felt that I was beginning to get things under control.

If I may shift forward a couple of years, printed a couple of paragraphs below is the letter I received after my routine check-up in early 2014. Again, I stress the Doctors words, that this route was working for me. The emphasis on the 'me'. My doctor is not suggesting that the route I chose would be right for others. The scientific evidence simply does not support such a conclusion. (Not least, because the scientific evidence has only been thinly researched; there is more profit in a cancer drug than a natural remedy we can find on the supermarket shelves. If, that is, such a cure does in fact exist.)

Nevertheless, you can imagine my delight at receiving acknowledgement of the decisions I had taken.

I need to stress once more, the route I took was working for me. It might not work for other people. The advice we receive from our oncologists is crucial to consider and, in most cases, follow. For example, we should always request a second opinion if the guidance we are given seems wrong, or not matched to our own circumstances. However, I suppose that the conclusion to draw from my own experience is that there is much to be gained – certainly psychologically and very probably physically – from taking charge of our cancer. Even if that taking charge involves doing no more than following the instructions of the specialist teams looking after us. Becoming pro-active rather that reactive is not a cure for cancer. If only it was. But it helps us to feel better, to feel in control. There is much to be said for being in that state.

It was in January that I came across a treatment which is sometimes known as metabolic therapy. This involves, believe it or not, consuming apricot seeds. I was very dubious. Who would not be? Getting at the seeds involves splitting the stone and removing the seeds from inside.

In fact, during my research, I learned of the Hunza tribe. These people come from the Hunza valley in Pakistan. They first came to prominence in the 1930s, when a Major in the Indian Medical Service, Sir Robert McCarrison, wrote about them. It seemed that they enjoyed near perfect health, with none of the ills of the West – obesity, heart attack, diabetes or cancer.

Then, in the 1950s, Dr Ernest Krebs, a biochemist seeking knowledge about cancer, discovered the writings and investigated further. It turned out that the Hunzas were active people, nomadic and herders of animals. They ate a healthy diet, with only a small amount of meat, raw milk and lots of vegetables.

Dr Krebs discovered, they ate huge amounts of apricot seeds. Within these humble foods is the active agent, a glucoside called amygdalin. It seemed, to Krebs back in the day, that amygdalin caused tumours to be destroyed.

Copy of my letter from the hospital following my January 2014 visit. Fortunately, matters appear to be looking up.

This entered the western market as 'Vitamin B17' or laetrile. It is especially effective in treating breast cancer, according to the website 'abukhadeejah.com'. However, it is not approved in the US. So while it is always important to take medical advice, working with a qualified healthcare practitioner, it does seem as though there is some evidence for the benefits of apricot seeds. Certainly, it is believed that they have formed a part of healing and healthcare regime for thousands of years.

But like so many other potentially beneficial natural products, apricot seeds have received a lot of bad press. Is the west missing out on a potentially very beneficial supplement? We need scientists to find out, and for that, somebody needs to come up with funding.

While I was drinking far more carrot juice than most people and literally turning orange, and tripling the recommended consumption of black seed oil, these are accepted supplements. The oil is less well known than carrot juice, but this is considered a cleanser for the body, the juice detoxifying the poisons that build up inside of people.

It is worth spending a short time examining the value of black seed oil as a supplement to our diet, because it is an oil that will be less well known by many readers. Once more, the origins of my consumption came from my religion. Cancer does this to us. It makes us revisit our spirituality. Inevitably, we find ourselves asking 'Why me?'; if as a cancer sufferer, or somebody close to one who has just been diagnosed with the condition, we cannot find faith within ourselves to provide succour in our distress, then many counsellors are trained in helping us to come to terms, mentally, with the shock of diagnosis. At least, as far as anyone ever can come to terms with such news. Spirituality takes many forms, and we find it in many ways. Often, we rekindle it through our religion, perhaps in consultation with our religious leaders. We might find it through mindfulness activities such as meditation, through good gestures such as helping others. We might find it in nature, or in our families. Wherever it comes from, our spirituality will become a comfort to us in the most difficult hours.

Mine came from my religion. Among the foodstuffs advocated by the Prophet (PBUH) is black seed oil. The Prophet (PBUH) said "Blackseed oil was the cure to all disease but death." Without that spiritual link, I may not have taken it, or I may have started its consumption too late, rather than at the first sign of the return of my cancer.

Many readers may know black seed oil better by its other name, black cumin. Its seeds come from the nigella sativa plant, which is in turn best known as the fennel flower. The seeds themselves, as well as the oil which can be pressed from them, is, like honey, a mainstay of traditional medicines from many cultures. It has been used for centuries – at least 1400 years. It is thought to have helped to have countered many diseases over time. Including cancer.

Unfortunately, and it is hard to know exactly why, trials of the natural medicine in human cancer are notably lacking. However, a study published in 2010, in the Oncology Letters medical publication demonstrated excellent results in rats. It was found that two daily doses of the oil, in its crude, extra virgin form, reduced cancers even in doses as small as 50mg per kg of bodyweight in the rodents. In particular, the study found, the oil was effective in inhibiting the growth of cancer tumours in lungs, the oesophagus, the stomach and the colon of rats. This led the study to conclude that black seed oil has carcino-preventative and chemo-preventative traits, with the potential that these could also apply in humans. Although, of course, studies would need to be undertaken. The study also theorised that black seed oil, taken in the early stages of cancer, could help to reduce the need for chemotherapy because it would suppress the spread of cancer cells.

The 2010 study was not alone in highlighting the potential for beneficial use of black seed oil in the treatment of cancer. In 2007 details were published in the Brazil Journal of Medical and Biological Research which suggested that black seed oil could be a supplement worth further investigation in the treatment of cancer in humans. Here, scientists induced tumours in rats and analysed the extent to which black seed oil limited their growth. In order to carry out their experiment, the researchers injected the oil into the cancer infused rats for thirty days, while the control group were left untreated. At the end of the thirty-day trial, the tumours in the control group averaged two and a half centimetres, whilst those in the treated rats averaged just one fifth of a centimetre. It seems compelling evidence that the value of black seed oil as a part of a range of remedies for addressing cancer should be advanced.

We know that the active compound in black seed oil, when it comes to its medicinal benefits, is thymoquinone. Notwithstanding that, there are more than a hundred different elements in black seed oil. One of them is nigellone, which two Egyptian researchers, Mahfouz and El-Dakhakhny, isolated as being beneficial to health as early as 1959. Nigellone is particularly beneficial in treating respiratory diseases. It is also an antihistamine, which makes it particularly attractive to allergy sufferers. Black seed oil also works as a handy anti-toxin, and it is believed to help regulate cholesterol and improve blood circulation.

Nevertheless, when it comes to cancer treatment, it is thymoquinone which may offer the best benefits towards treating the tumours which proliferate. In one of the extremely few tests into human cancers, during 2008 scientists carried out a lab-based study in which they injected low dose thymoquinone into cancerous tumours from a human prostrate. The tests were carried out with the tumours based in a petri dish, rather than inside the body. However, the tests were successful. The tumour stopped growing, no new blood vessels formed in them, and they stopped reproducing. There were no observable side effects. The research was published in Molecular Cancer Therapeutics and the study's conclusion was that thymoquinone stops tumour growth in humans and could have potential as a treatment for cancer.

It does really seem that taking black seed oil does no harm, at the very least. That is the first premise of any treatment, that it should do no more harm than the condition it is seeking to tackle. In all probability, the oil might offer considerable benefits, at least in some types of cancer. It certainly seems as though there are grounds for further research. It might seem strange that such knowledge is yet to be sought.

Except that it has. In 2011 an article was published in the American Journal of Chinese Medicine which demonstrated that there have been numerous studies into the side effects of taking black seed oil or thymoquinone. The studies looked at the supplements taken orally, and on a long-term basis. None were discovered. So, we see, there is a degree of positive scientific evidence behind the medicinal benefits of black seed oil. It is just that we have to dig hard to find it. However, there is a caveat associated with this herbal medicine. With larger doses (tests were at 2 g per kg of weight) taken daily, there was some evidence of liver and kidney damage in rats. It may therefore be the case that higher doses are unsafe in humans. Further, the possibility remains (because it hasn't been ruled out) that black seed oil may interact with other drugs a patient is taking. In turn, this may lead to harmful side effects.

Black seed oil has worked superbly for me, but I advise with the strongest intent that before taking this supplement, cancer sufferers should consult their doctor.

So, carrot juice, honey and, to a lesser extent, black seed oil are each mainstays of natural, alternative medicines. Apricot seeds are a different matter. Until reading about their health-giving benefits, I had never come across anybody consuming these. I did not even know that they could be eaten. But suffering from cancer heightens the brain. I became almost zealous about this possible aid to my fight. I read everything I could find on the subject, and decided that the results and evidence, some of which was anecdotal, certainly made trying out the therapy worthwhile. As is my wont, once I committed to the treatment, I really gave it my all, apricot seed therapy also known as metabolic therapy. I was soon consuming up to thirty or forty seeds a day, taking five or six every two to three hours. My reading also advocated the use of vitamin C tablets (2000mg), adding zinc to my diet (via 17mg pills) and taking pancreatic enzyme tablets.

It is hard to convey the confused state of my mental health at this point. I was virtually three months into my self-designed treatments. There was this constant nagging in my mind that I might have made the worst kind of mistake. One that would literally kill me. What I really lacked was reassurance. Nobody I could speak to could tell me that I was doing the right thing. Because, as we have said again and again, and will say once more here, cancer is unique to each and every sufferer. The individuality of my version of the disease was compounded by the fact that my treatment was unique as well. Everybody close to me, with the best will in the world, advised me to find the added assurance of what a hospital could offer. To go back to my oncology team and tell them to get to work.

As they rightly said, I could not see into my body. Maybe tumours were already spreading into my lungs, spreading throughout my body and attacking my essential organs. I would not know; the pain of cancer is one that only a cancer patient can relate to.

'Stop messing about, get to hospital and get yourself checked,' the message was consistent. I have no doubt that I possess a rebellious personality. I would not re-take my A levels at Camp Hill school, choosing instead a rough college with a reputation many leagues below the school with its national reputation for academic excellence. That was a risk. I gave up my first dabble into law to try my hand at business; that was an (expensive) risk. But risk taking is generally seen as an admirable quality. Plain stupidity is not. The problem is, there is a very narrow divide between the two, and I was far from sure on which side of the line I was residing.

Yet…yet…physically I did not feel too bad; there was no evidence that my condition was deteriorating. Mentally, despite the worries, I felt good that I had taken control, was taking charge of defeating the colonising aliens inside my body. Maybe, perhaps, possibly… I was doing the right thing.

Still I stuck with my extreme diet. The apricot seeds were the hardest. They were so bitter. The best way to describe them is as a kind of unsweetened, highly sharp, marzipan. I had given up all meat, including chicken. Breakfast would consist of grapes with seeds, topped with chunks of papaya and pineapple. I read somewhere that the hard core of a pineapple could lead to the withering of cancer cells as it contained something called bromelain, so I did not just eat the succulent outer flesh of the spiky fruit, but the tough inner block as well. I continued to avoid sugar – again from the advice my research was offering – holding to the belief that to deprive my body of sugar, particularly the processed sugars that come in chunky white packets, I would starve the cancer cells of oxygen, adding to their decline.

For two years I stuck to the diet: black seed oil and carrot juice – both in copious quantities – three times a day. Copious relative to the recommended amounts. I avoided sugar and managed my diet through fruit and vegetables.

Dear ████████████

Altaf Hussain, DOB 13/09/1977, ███████████████████

Clinic attendance: 9 July 2014   Clinic: FUCLIHAE

Diagnosis: Hodgkin's disease diagnosed 2001
Treated with ChlVPP/PABLOE in the LY09 trial
Relapsed in December 2011 with isolated disease in the neck confirmed on PET scan but declined any treatment
No further progression clinically
Last PET scan April 2012 positive

Drugs prescribed at clinic: **Nil**

Haemoglobin 170 g/L   WBC 5.18 x 10⁹/l   Neutrophils 1.63 x 10⁹/l   Platelets 204 x 10⁹/l

This gentleman is well without any B symptoms per se. He does get the odd drenching night sweat but it is very occasional about once every two months.

On examination today there are some minor but tiny less than 1 cm lymph nodes within the neck. There is no palpable disease anywhere.

He remains exceptionally well working full time. Therefore, we will see him again in six months' time. Should any problems arise in the future we will always be happy to see him sooner.

Kind regards
Yours sincerely

████████

Consultant Haematologist

Letter from the hospital after my July 2014 check up. Matters are looking up, and I can see some light, but I am not yet clear of the woods.

Papaya and pineapple continued to feature consistently in my daily meals. I always treated myself with the full awareness of my oncologist, who was in many ways supportive of my offbeat approach to tackling my cancer. However, I did rub up against the blunt wall of NHS administration. I do understand that cancer treatment is very expensive. I do get that budgets are tight, and it is important that priorities are established. But I was saving my hospital a fortune by refusing chemotherapy or radiotherapy. There was one thing that they could have done which would have helped my anxiety. That was to offer me a scan.

But, since I declined chemotherapy it was as though, at an administrative level, they washed their hands of me. Do as we say, or face the consequences seemed to be the line these ivory tower housed faceless ones were determined to deliver. There were times when it felt as though this was a kind of narrow-vision arrogance, an idea that only they knew what was best for me. Not the practitioners, note – whilst I am sure that these experts must have worried that I declined more traditional treatments, they remained supportive. But the money men – or women – who to my mind, did not have the slightest idea what treatment suited me best.

So, with no scans available to tell me if my diet-based regime was working at reducing the tumours proliferating on my inside, I was left to employ other methods. Blunt ones. My belief in myself could not be supported by science, because I dared to take responsibility for my own well-being, but there were other clues. I was able to work full time; I was able to play football and tennis, go to the gym and even climb mountains. Compare that to the decimation of my body and will the first time, when chemotherapy put the cancer into remission, but knocked me out for six months in the process. To all intents and purposes, I was fit and healthy. Just a fit and healthy man with cancer.

Allow me to take a turn back in time, back to December 28th, 2011. Christmas time seems to feature prominently in my cancer diagnoses. This was the day that I had the results of my biopsy. The news that my Hodgkin's lymphoma had returned seemed, on the surface, to hit my father hardest. He was devastated, the sadness written across his face. I think he genuinely believed that, this time, all hope was gone. My mum tried to be stronger.

'Whatever Allah wills,' she said. Mum knows best. Always.

Sentence Served

7th August 2012

A transcript of the letter from my Consultant Haematology Team at Heartlands

It was a pleasure to see your pleasant patient Altaf in the lymphoma clinic today. I am delighted to know he is generally well in himself apart from symptoms of indigestion with epigastric discomfort. He denied any new lymphadenopathy of B symptoms.

On clinical examination there is no palpable lymph adenopathy in the cervical, axillary or inguinal region. Abdominal examination did not reveal any palpable hepatosplenomegaly but there is minimal tenderness in the epigastric region.

In view of his history of indigestion it is prudent to proceed with upper GI endoscopy. Altaf want to think about it before proceeding with upper GI endoscopy. I have asked Altaf to either contact you or me if he decides to proceed with upper GI endoscopy. I shall review him in 4 months' time. Altaf is aware to seek medical opinion urgently if there is any lymphadenopathy or drenching night sweats. I shall keep you updated with his progress.

For more than two years, I kept up the daily regime of diet-based treatment which, as far as I could tell, was tackling my cancer effectively. I am not going to say it was easy; I was working full time as a lawyer as well as running my own law firm. There were setbacks, such as the suggestion that I needed an endoscopy, as shown in the transcript on the previous page. But to my mind there were few options. Basically, I had to cope, or I could die. I think that it was about 2014 that I started to relax.

Today I am here, fit and well, nine years after that second attack, and two decades after the first, is, I believe testament to the human spirit. I am not saying that we can will ourselves to live. The opposite of that implies that those who die lacked the strength of spirit to survive. To even conceive of such a thought is disrespectful to the suffering those victims, and their families, endured. What I am saying is that with strength of spirit, commitment to a therapy and determination to see it through, we can overcome terrible adversity.

Sometimes, even that is not enough. But by becoming active in our own treatment of this despicable disease we increase our chances of defeating it. I am not suggesting that I have found a cure for cancer, but instead that, with our doctor's advice and support, combinations of natural nutritional sources, plus adherence to a strict and healthy diet could help.

Of course, we are all different, and I cannot stress often enough that everybody's individual experience of cancer, with all its myriad columns of variations and variables, is unique to them. What worked for me may not work for others.

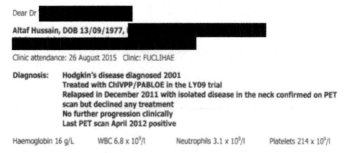

Dear Dr ████████████

Altaf Hussain, DOB 13/09/1977, ████████████████

Clinic attendance: 26 August 2015 Clinic: FUCLIHAE

Diagnosis: **Hodgkin's disease diagnosed 2001**
Treated with ChlVPP/PABLOE in the LY09 trial
Relapsed in December 2011 with isolated disease in the neck confirmed on PET scan but declined any treatment
No further progression clinically
Last PET scan April 2012 positive

Haemoglobin 16 g/L   WBC 6.8 x 10^9/l   Neutrophils 3.1 x 10^9/l   Platelets 214 x 10^9/l

It was a pleasure to see Mr Hussain in today's outpatient clinic. His condition remains stable. He has a small lymph node palpable in the neck, but no other areas of lymphadenopathy or hepatosplenomegaly. He denies any B symptoms and we will see him back in our clinic in six months time.

An update from September 2015. Still all ok.

I must not downplay the role of my oncologist and their team in holding the upper hand in my battle with cancer. That I chose my own route, trusting to diet and a positive outlook, is not to suggest that the support I received from my hospital was not crucial to my on-going health.   From 2011 to 2014 I would go to the hospital every six months. There I would be weighed. I lost weight, but I am sure that this was due to my strict and healthy diet, rather than because of my cancer. Since I could not be scanned, due to the administrators' decision, I used this as one of the indicators of my health. If the cancer was not showing, I deduced, the chances were that it was receding. The nurse would do a blood test, and the doctors at the hospital would be more and more amazed at what I had achieved. They saw me shrink the tumours in my neck.

After about five years of this six-monthly regime, I discharged myself from the hospital. I decided that I did not need testing, that what was being measured I could do myself, and that the mental stress of these visits, although time gradually reduced it, were more damaging to my mental health than the benefits they offered to my physical well-being. My family disagreed with my decision. I cannot blame them for that. Their interest was always in me, and what set of actions would do most to ensure that I survived the cancer. However, I decided that I had to honour the commitment I had made to tackling this disease myself. My measures of the state of my cancer would be simple. Could I walk? Could I run?

Yet, for all these apparently determined decisions, I am not going to pretend that my anxiety did not remain. I could push it away, lock it in a cupboard in my mind, but it had – and still has – a way of creeping out when I least expect it. What if the cancer has not gone away, but is just biding its time? What if my decision to control this disease myself was wrong? What if I get a third bout of the disease? They are questions that linger. To be honest, I am not sure that they will ever be answered or go fully away.

For all this, I am proud of what I achieved. I hold on to the belief that my cancer was beaten largely by the careful diet I put into my body. For this reason, I continue to take the relevant foodstuff. My diet is not as good as it was, but I still watch it, and from time to time will return to the strict days, as though to give myself a boost of the healthy stuff and a rest from the less nutritious intake which is now such an omnipresent, although destructive, part of western diet. Although I no longer swallow apricot seeds as thought they were gulps of air – to me, particularly noxious gulps of air – I still continue to take them from time to time. Around once a week I will consume a glass of carrot juice, laced with black seed oil. I regard these routines as like the servicing of a car. I probably don't need them, but by keeping up their consumption I am, I hope, staving off trouble in the future.

Cancer charities do a wonderful job, but I really wish they would sponsor more research into the power of diet. There is so little of this. I am not saying it is a miracle cure to cancer. Of course not. But if it helps even one person, surely the effort is worthwhile. I can't help but believe that many more than one person would benefit from proper research into the power of diet. Of course, we live in a commercial world. There is more money in chemical treatments than natural ones.

I understand that, although do not agree with it. But that is where charities could step in. Use more of their money to seek treatments from what we already have, not what the human race can create.

I am not complaining, because I enjoy it very much. But being chairman of an international law firm in the UK, is a stressful job. I am constantly involved in challenging cases across the globe. It is my competitive nature – dating back to my younger days on the football pitches at school or in the park – to want to win. That competitive spirit combined with the sense of justice I still hold dear. That does not show itself through punching a bully anymore, but by seeking truth and justice through legal process. So, each case is, in its own way, something taxing. This is possibly not the best way to live when the risk that a life-threatening serious illness could return at any moment. But we are what we are. We deal with challenges as we see fit.

In fact, getting back to normal (or, to quote the oft-used Covid 19 induced cliché, the 'new normal') can be one of the bigger challenges for many cancer sufferers. I suspect that those feelings I endured when I made the decision to turn down chemotherapy, and treat myself, are shared with others who have followed the more orthodox route, with success. In both cases, the weekly, then monthly, visits to hospital suddenly cease. There might now be six months between appointments. That is a long time to wait nervously for the reassurance that everything is still OK. Without warning, the cancer team who have supported us, offering their expert opinions and comforting experience are gone. They move on to other patients, but we remain with our anxieties. Meanwhile, for the cancer patient, it is not unusual to sense a kind of loss that we no longer see these people on a regular basis.

Re-joining our family is no easy thing, either. Roles change, our natural place might have been usurped by others, and that is their 'new normal'. It can be hard, and just as cancer knocks our confidence in ourselves, we may find it hard to say how we are thinking. We will have that lurking sense that people judge us:

'He's recovered from cancer; he should be grateful and accept everything he has...'

Not ill meant, but just not understanding that even when we are cured of the disease, fear inevitably remains, at least to some extent. We may worry that we will hurt the feelings of people who have helped us, but now replaced us. We are thrown into a difficult, challenging balancing act in our social arrangements, there is no getting away from that.

And suddenly we have time. No longer is every waking moment (and many sleeping ones, as well) spent either enduring the latest wave of treatment, recovering from it or anticipating the next one. We now have the chance to reflect. Cancer certainly adds experience to our personalities, but it also takes away other opportunities. We may find that we have missed that promotion at work which, had we been well, we would have sought; that we have lost a vital year or two of our children's or grandchildren's upbringing, that we have not had enough quality time to spend with family – our parents, siblings as well as our spouse and children.

Now we have time to reflect on these losses. It is quite understandable and completely acceptable to suddenly become very angry. Or sad. Or scared. We are all different. Cancer affects us in different ways. Unless we have experienced it, we cannot begin to imagine what the disease does to us. These are all points I have already made. All points that still apply. Our loved ones might move on, relieved that we seem to be in remission, seem to have recovered. It could well take us longer. In fact, we will never be quite the same again.

There are bodily changes as well. I have already explained that I am somehow less physically strong than I used to be; that I look different. Not hugely so, but enough to be reminded every time I look in a mirror. This is reinforced every time I meet an acquaintance I have not seen in a while.

'You're looking well...' they smile, before pausing on the unsaid part, '...considering you've had cancer.'

Those words might not be voiced, but they are implied. Not nastily, or critically. The opposite, in fact. Still though a reminder that I am not quite the person I was.

It is usual as well to experience intense – worrying, even – tiredness when we see the end of our cancer treatment. Firstly, the lingering side effects of the treatment we have undergone remain in our bodies for a while, but more than that suddenly the stress that has held us tight for so long goes. We are not used to relaxing; we are not used to making decisions free from the restraints cancer applies. People view us differently; no longer are we 'suffering from cancer' but we become 'cancer survivors', a subtle change in outlook which can take some getting used to.

Facing these feelings is another task cancer inflicts upon us. But as with the shocks to our emotional and physical state that being diagnosed with cancer brings, so too we must accept these feelings. We should honour them, respect them, embrace them. Only then can we pack them away.

I do believe that my own successful battle was down more than any other factor to the changes to my diet, the poisons I stopped consuming and the de-toxifying natural foodstuffs and supplements I began to take. But I also believe that being positive in deciding to tackle the disease played a very, very significant part in my recovery.

Yet, again, we run the risk of encountering the well-meant but not apposite views of those who do not really understand what we have been through, and what we fear we may face again. The importance of a positive attitude is one of the definers of the early part of the 21st century. I am not saying it is not important, but as with so much else, how we define our own positive outlook is down to us. It is not for others to impose their own viewpoints on us. Especially when we are vulnerable. In writing this book I wanted to share my story; I hope it will help readers in coming to terms with their own cancer, or that in a loved one, or even in the fear of getting cancer, something we all find lurking deep inside of us. But what worked for me, literally did just that. It worked for me; it doesn't mean it will work for others. It might. It might not.

So, I find those who 'know best' particularly irksome. Coping with cancer is down to the sufferer; all that others can do is offer as much education for those with the disease to access as they can. I fear that it is one of the biggest dangers, and biggest barriers, to a full mental (and therefore, physical) recovery that sufferers can face that they feel they must appear positive. They should be constantly upbeat around others, dismissing their own genuine and completely understandable feelings. That they should be grateful for a recovery. (Which is like being grateful that the burglar who stole almost everything of value from our house at least decided to leave behind our TV).

Please, be aware that there is absolutely zero evidence that a positive mindset will cure cancer; that it will stop it from coming back. Or, conversely, that a return of a cancer is the result of a negative outlook or thoughts. Positivity can make us *feel* better, and that brings many additional benefits. However, *such positivity is our own, individual version of thought*. Adopting somebody else's positivity when we are not comfortable with it, or it stops us expressing our true emotions because of guilt or concern that we will make people worried or angry, really is not helping us. We should be aware of giving way to the positive attitude compulsives, the keep smiling conspiracists. We must not allow them to prevent us from telling our family, friends, spouses, colleagues and medical team how we really feel. Or, most importantly of all, allow them to stop us being honest towards our own feelings, however good or bad they might be.

Having lived through cancer, or any major illness for that matter, can make us ultra-sensitive to our bodies. While the doctor will have confirmed that the cancer is gone, small aches and pains can take on magnified importance in our minds. We question ourselves. 'Will I fall foul of the disease once more? What is the likelihood of a return, and how will I know if the cancer has invaded my body again? What will I do if I do receive another attack?' The prospect of going through the worry, the pain, the uncertainty once more can erode even the most robust consciousness. Always, niggling away like waves wearing away the coastline is the negative thought that, yes, the disease will return. I just don't know when.

All that I can offer, having been through this twice now, is that over time the fear diminishes. We learn to live with the anxiety. Even so, certain triggers can set the mind running once more. Hospital check-ups and anniversaries of key dates can be the worst. Often, we will have established support groups during our illness. These will sometimes contain other cancer victims and learning that one of these new friends has had a relapse frequently leads to the sense that we are on borrowed time ourselves. Both new and a return of previous symptoms inevitably set our minds running towards what these signs might represent. Remember – cancer changes us. It makes us stronger, true. But it also makes us more vulnerable.

But despite these worries there is plenty that we can do to make our consciousness more robust against these psychological pits. Here are some ideas that I use myself, and which I have gathered through my reading of the subject and discussions with others. As with all suggestions, it is about finding what each of us individually discovers will help to reduce our anxiety.

Control what we can, accept what we can't: If we study the subject, read about what other people have tried to stop their cancer returning, we feel in control. That state of mind is a good way to restrict anxiety. However, while we can stay fit, and avoid obvious carcinogenic substances, we must also understand that if the cancer is going to return, then it will. If we accept that fact, it becomes easier to cope with it.

Little techniques can help us regain control. Setting up a daily schedule works for some people, Routine is reassuring. Accept that these negative thoughts will enter our mind from time to time. Recognise when they arrive and do something active to distract our mind away from them.

I think it has been a recurring theme throughout this book that when we accept that having cancer really isn't very pleasant, it immediately becomes less of a threat, less of a worry, less of a control on our lives. Of course, it remains a danger, and we will be concerned about that. It will impact on what we can do, both during treatment and after it has been sent on its way. But knowledge is power, and acceptance is the first step towards accommodating the situation in which we are required to live.

Live in the present: The past is a hard time for cancer survivors, memories are unpleasant; the future holds uncertainty for everybody. But the now is something we can more easily control. We can practice throwing out worries about what is going to happen to us, or painful memories about what we have been through by learning what makes us feel at peace. It might be something like listening to music, going for a walk, picking up a book, doing some baking or involving ourselves in other hobbies. Even throwing ourselves into our work. Then, when we feel ourselves drifting out of the now, we can grab hold of that tool which brings us peace, and by applying it we will feel better.

Give ourselves a chance: There is no question that being physically as fit as we can be, eating a healthy diet, cutting down on alcohol consumption and stopping smoking are all health based life decisions we can take, and which can reduce our likelihood of both our cancer returning and, for our friends and family, stopping it from occurring in the first place.

If we are genetically programmed to suffer from cancer, then certainly with where science stands at the moment, we may well get it. But surely anything that reduces the odds of the horror of cancer returning is a price worth paying. A price that comes with the added bonus that we look better and feel better in ourselves.

Achieving that state of physical health might not be as daunting as it appears. For those that find it difficult, whose personalities are often compulsive or who simply do not enjoy exercise (and why should everybody?), the secret is to set small, achievable targets. Take the stairs rather than the lift at work. Walk rather than drive to the local shop. Make sure that we do not have chocolate in the house. Instead, ensure that we always have fruit and nuts available.

Cook a meal rather than buy a processed dish or a takeaway. Not every day, but more often. Aim to cut down smoking slowly, until we no longer crave the poisons which come from the weed. Walk for twenty minutes a day. Then, slowly, increase the amount. Marginal gains, easily achieved. Keep an eye out for latest research information that might be of benefit to us.

For example, there is a study called HITS being undertaken at Nottingham University at present. HITS is a high intensity training programme which could be ideal for those looking to clear health threatening conditions such as diabetes and obesity, which can increase our chances of getting cancer, and limit our ability to fight the disease.

HITS sounds ideal for those who simply loathe regular exercise, for the surprisingly high figure (about a fifth of people) who gain minimal benefit from traditional exercise or those who cannot jog because of other ailments.

HITS should only be undertaken after consultation with our doctor, because strain on the heart can be caused, but if the go ahead is given it fundamentally features three twenty second bursts of full on, high intensity activity three times a week. Three minutes every seven days. Anybody can find that minimal amount of time. Preliminary studies suggest that the training educates the body to increase metabolism and burn fat. Perfect for the people who, for whatever reason, get little from traditional exercise regimes, or who simply hate exercise.

I am fortunate in that I have always loved sport and exercise. Not everybody feels the same way.

Accept Our Fears: It is one of those unfortunate accepted beliefs that holding fear can make us feel weak. It tells us that we are lack inner strength. This is not the case. Everybody holds fear about something or other. Because of our previous cancer, we are especially prone to worries and anxieties. It is as it is. We should not judge ourselves because of this. Instead, we should practise mindfulness techniques which help us to let go of our fears. Meditation, yoga, reading, visualising our fears floating away, putting our faith in our spiritual beliefs. All are methods we can try to help us to learn to live with fear, to accept that this is something which will enter into our minds on occasion. At the same time, these techniques will help us to prevent fears from dominating our consciousness.

Making use of friends and counsellors to whom we can verbalise our fears is also a good idea. Just talking through our worries can help us to resolve them. It can sometimes be hard to do this with people to whom we are close. That is where the benefit of approaching an objective counsellor, a person we will only meet within a professional context, can be a useful activity.

A word about counsellors. The term is generic for a number of levels of qualification. The most highly trained of these professionals will hold a Master's degree in the subject and will have studied for perhaps two years to get their initial qualification, whilst undertaking regular training to keep them fresh and up to date once in the workplace. On the other hand, I saw an advert from the bargain retailer Wowcher recently, offering a counselling course for £12. Apparently, this led to a level three qualification, whatever that might mean. People with either of those extreme levels of expertise can quite legitimately call themselves a counsellor. Naturally, simply studying for a long period at a high standard does not automatically make a person a better counsellor, but it is likely to mean that their understanding of the workings of the mind is stronger, and the techniques they can apply towards helping us more nuanced and researched. Hiring a counsellor is not cheap, at the time of writing, many more highly qualified practitioners will charge between £40 and £60 per hour for their services, more in some cases.

However, it is also true that most counsellors also offer a pro bono service, often through a separate charity. A chat with our GP or a visit to our local civic centre can point us towards professionals working on a voluntary basis.

Those who have successfully tackled alcoholism usually refer to themselves as recovering alcoholics. The phrase helps them to recognise that they can succumb to the disease once more at any time. We are recovering cancer sufferers; recognising that the possibility exists that we can fall to the disease again helps us to take the actions to mitigate against that and makes the possibility of it easier to manage. At the same time, we know what to look for, often we will have the benefit of regular check-ups. Anybody can get cancer, and we are in the fortunate position of knowing how to recognise symptoms, spotting signs early, with all the benefits that can bring.

I am nine years clear from my second bout of the disease. It may return once more; I hope it does not. That is the life I, and the millions like me, live. I would prefer not to have the cloud always just there, these days existing only on the horizon, but nevertheless still dark and threatening. A storm which will probably bypass me by many miles but which, I know, could be heading slowly in my direction; to suddenly pour down on me when I least expect it. Over time I have learned not to look at those clouds, and although every day I am faced with glimpses of this distant danger – the scar on my neck, my physical weakness, the diet I eat – I can live with it.

I have a close and caring family, a good circle of loyal friends, an interesting and successful career and a loving wife. I am not going to let cancer get in the way of enjoying such a great life.

Epilogue – My Diet for Life

When the oncologist had confirmed my cancer had returned in January of 2012 I was devastated.

I didn't know what to do. Dad was upset. Mum was shocked. I remember looking into the sky many times asking for help from God. No solution offered itself to me, but I was determined that there were no circumstances whereby I would put chemotherapy back into my body.

Some of the articles I read suggested combining grape juice with blackseed oil, but more went for the carrot juice and blacksee oil route. In the end, really for no reason other than it appeared more regularly, I went for that latter option.

That first sight of the return of my cancer was late in 2011 – I knew before the diagnosis; call it instinct, gut feeling, experience, fatalism…whatever. I knew that it was back. From that moment my life seemed consumed by reading and juicing. Black seed oil three times a day. By the following February I could see that the tumour on my neck was not growing. The Prophet Muhammed (PBUH) said: 'Blackseed oil was the cure to all disease but death.' As a Muslim, I have complete faith in the word of the high figure of the Islamic world.

However, despite this there was not any scientific evidence for the benefits of mixing carrot juice with blackseed oil in terms of tackling Hodgkin's lymphoma. There still is not. The only evidence was anecdotal. I was sceptical about the chances of success at first but stuck with it. Meanwhile, friends Dr Hak and clinical research pharmacist Rez were advocating chemotherapy.

I went against all my friends, family and, I have to say, the advice of some expert doctors.

I then discovered apricot seed therapy, which is also known as metabolic therapy. This is really very controversial. It was first discovered by a Dr Krebs and then his son a Dr Krebs Jnr. The FDA states that if we eat too many seeds it can lead to cyanide poisoning. I must admit to becoming scared by these articles. I was terrified, I even contacted a member of a cult in the United States, an extreme Christian guy. His advice was 'By the blood of Jesus Christ this will work.'

I wasn't convinced, not yet, and was still worried. But not as much as by the prospect of either chemotherapy, or death. I just went for it in the end.

This is what my diet became, for more than two years. I was never overly heavy but lost nearly one and a half stones in weight over this time. Nowadays I still eat healthily, and from time to time return to an abbreviated version of my diet. Below is a summary of my personal treatment which I did religiously for two years.

Apricot Seeds

I ate 30-40 apricot seeds per day, 6 at a time every few hours. Fortunately, I did not succumb to cyanide poisoning, although the bitter almond taste of the seeds was unpleasant, at least to me. I did notice a little rash and you can feel cold as they lower your blood pressure. Apparently, it is the amagdyline in the apricot seeds which is what makes them effective against cancer cells.

Pineapple

The hard core of this sumptuous fruit is particularly beneficial. It contains bromelain, which is believed by some to be very good at attacking and destroying cancer cells. I ate pineapple on a daily basis.

Papaya

I admit that quite quickly I became sick to death of this fruit as I would eat large amounts everyday. I read It contains vitamins, that help weaken cancer cells.

Zinc

I took a 17 mg tablet daily, but also ate foods high in zinc such as avocado, pumpkin, sunflower and sesame seeds. Zinc helps transport vitamins around the body.

Vitamin C

I also took vitamin C as a supplement, consuming a 2000mg tablet each day. With all the fruit and vegetables I was consuming, I was really knocking back the Vitamin C. The idea is to boost the immune system to the max.

Pancreatic Enzyme Tablets

Some of the ingredients in these tablets mirrored what I was consuming through eating the papaya and pineapple. I took two to four Pancreatic Enzyme tablets each day.

Milk Thistle in Green Tea

I did not mention this in the main body of the book. However, milk thistle is believed to be good for the liver, and many cancer patients suffer from impaired liver function. Green tea is generally recognised as containing anti-toxin qualities; it is also pleasant to drink!

My friend Asif came round in April 2012 to my house, he told me it was good for the liver. I took it every day with green tea.

Blackseed Oil with Carrot Juice

I would drink 3 cups of carrot juice a day, one in the morning, one for lunch and one in the evening, each time I would add a teaspoon of blackseed oil.

Brazil Nuts

I read that if I ate brazil nuts, I could rid my body of toxins. I would eat 3-4 a day.

My diet contained no sugar or meat, other than occasionally a little fish with rice or bread when I felt really hungry. I consumed almost exclusively fruit, vegetables and seeds.

I rubbed down my tumours with blackseed oil, while reciting Sura Fatiha from The Holy Quran,

7 or 11 times every day, asking Allah to cure me of cancer.

As I have said many times through this book, I am making no claims at all that this approach would work for anybody else.

But thank goodness, it worked for me.

If you enjoyed reading my book, would you mind taking a minute to write a review? Even a short review helps, and it would mean a lot to me.

If you like you can follow me on TikTok @kungfulawyer, connect with me on LinkedIn, or Facebook.

For legal enquiries you can email me at altaf@addisonaaron.com

Best Regards

The Angel's Advocate

Heart of England Centre
for Haematology and Stem Cell Transplantation
Clinical Director   Tel: E-mail address

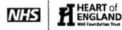

Birmingham Heartlands Hospital
Bordesley Green East
Bordesley Green
Birmingham B9 5SS

Tel: 0121 424 2000
Fax: 0121 766 7530

www.haematology-heartlands.nhs.uk

8 June 2016

Dear Dr Trent

Altaf Hussain,

Clinic attendance: 18 May 2016   Clinic: FUCLIHAE

Diagnosis: **Hodgkin's disease diagnosed 2001**
Treated with ChlVPP/PABLOE in the LY09 trial
Relapsed in December 2011 with isolated disease in the neck confirmed on PET scan but declined any treatment
No further progression clinically
Last PET scan April 2012 positive

Haemoglobin 171 g/L   WBC 6.5 x 10⁹/l   Neutrophils 2.5 x 10⁹/l   Platelets 207 x 10⁹/l

Mr Hussain remains very well. On examination the palpable lymph node was a 1 ½cm diameter node at the bottom of the left anterior cervical chain. This node appears to have been stable for several years. Mr Hussain would like to be discharged from the clinic, and that is ok with me. He knows to seek medical attention promptly if he has any problems that suggest a relapse of his Hodgkin's lymphoma.

Yours sincerely

Consultant Haematologist

c.c.   **CONFIDENTIAL**
MR A HUSSAIN

Awarded for excellence

Great news.

Printed in Great Britain
by Amazon